ESCHERICHIA COLI O157:H7
IN GROUND BEEF

Review of a Draft Risk Assessment

Committee on the Review of the USDA *E. coli* O157:H7
Farm-to-Table Process Risk Assessment

Board on Health Promotion and Disease Prevention
Food and Nutrition Board

INSTITUTE OF MEDICINE
OF THE NATIONAL ACADEMIES

THE NATIONAL ACADEMIES PRESS
Washington, D.C.
www.nap.edu

THE NATIONAL ACADEMIES PRESS • 500 FIFTH STREET, N.W. • Washington, DC 20001

NOTICE: The project that is the subject of this report was approved by the Governing Board of the National Research Council, whose members are drawn from the councils of the National Academy of Sciences, the National Academy of Engineering, and the Institute of Medicine. The members of the committee responsible for the report were chosen for their special competences and with regard for appropriate balance.

Support for this project was provided by the US Department of Agriculture. The views presented in this report are those of the Institute of Medicine Committee on the Review of the USDA *E. coli* O157:H7 Farm-to-Table Process Risk Assessment and are not necessarily those of the funding agencies.

International Standard Book No. 0-309-08627-2

Additional copies of this report are available for sale from the National Academies Press, 500 Fifth Street, N.W., Box 285, Washington, D.C. 20055; call (800) 624-6242 or (202) 334-3313 (in the Washington metropolitan area); Internet, http://www.nap.edu.

For more information about the Institute of Medicine, visit the IOM home page at: **www.iom.edu.**

Copyright 2002 by the National Academy of Sciences. All rights reserved.

Printed in the United States of America.

The serpent has been a symbol of long life, healing, and knowledge among almost all cultures and religions since the beginning of recorded history. The serpent adopted as a logotype by the Institute of Medicine is a relief carving from ancient Greece, now held by the Staatliche Museen in Berlin.

*"Knowing is not enough; we must apply.
Willing is not enough; we must do."*
—Goethe

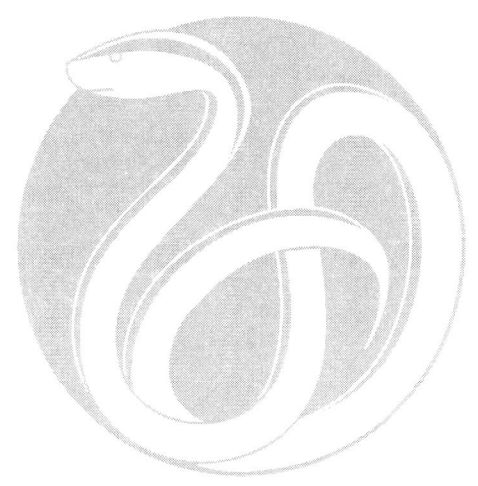

INSTITUTE OF MEDICINE
OF THE NATIONAL ACADEMIES

Shaping the Future for Health

THE NATIONAL ACADEMIES
Advisers to the Nation on Science, Engineering, and Medicine

The **National Academy of Sciences** is a private, nonprofit, self-perpetuating society of distinguished scholars engaged in scientific and engineering research, dedicated to the furtherance of science and technology and to their use for the general welfare. Upon the authority of the charter granted to it by the Congress in 1863, the Academy has a mandate that requires it to advise the federal government on scientific and technical matters. Dr. Bruce M. Alberts is president of the National Academy of Sciences.

The **National Academy of Engineering** was established in 1964, under the charter of the National Academy of Sciences, as a parallel organization of outstanding engineers. It is autonomous in its administration and in the selection of its members, sharing with the National Academy of Sciences the responsibility for advising the federal government. The National Academy of Engineering also sponsors engineering programs aimed at meeting national needs, encourages education and research, and recognizes the superior achievements of engineers. Dr. Wm. A. Wulf is president of the National Academy of Engineering.

The **Institute of Medicine** was established in 1970 by the National Academy of Sciences to secure the services of eminent members of appropriate professions in the examination of policy matters pertaining to the health of the public. The Institute acts under the responsibility given to the National Academy of Sciences by its congressional charter to be an adviser to the federal government and, upon its own initiative, to identify issues of medical care, research, and education. Dr. Harvey V. Fineberg is president of the Institute of Medicine.

The **National Research Council** was organized by the National Academy of Sciences in 1916 to associate the broad community of science and technology with the Academy's purposes of furthering knowledge and advising the federal government. Functioning in accordance with general policies determined by the Academy, the Council has become the principal operating agency of both the National Academy of Sciences and the National Academy of Engineering in providing services to the government, the public, and the scientific and engineering communities. The Council is administered jointly by both Academies and the Institute of Medicine. Dr. Bruce M. Alberts and Dr. Wm. A. Wulf are chair and vice chair, respectively, of the National Research Council

www.national-academies.org

COMMITTEE ON THE REVIEW OF THE USDA *E. COLI* O157:H7 FARM-TO-TABLE PROCESS RISK ASSESSMENT

Michael P. Doyle, PhD (Chair), Regents Professor of Food Microbiology and Director of the Center for Food Safety, University of Georgia, Griffin, Georgia

Scott Ferson, PhD, Senior Scientist and Vice President, Applied Biomathematics, Setauket, New York

Dale D. Hancock, DVM, MS, PhD, Professor and Epidemiologist, Field Disease Investigation Unit, Department of Veterinary Clinical Sciences, Washington State University, Pullman, Washington

Myron M. Levine, MD, DTPH, Professor and Director, University of Maryland School of Medicine, Center for Vaccine Development, Baltimore, Maryland

Greg Paoli, MASc, President, Decisionalysis Risk Consultants, Inc., Ottawa, Ontario

Barbara J. Peterson, PhD, MPH, Principal/Practice Director, Food and Chemicals Practice, Exponent, Washington, DC

John N. Sofos, PhD, Professor, Department of Animal Sciences, Colorado State University, Fort Collins, Colorado

Susan S. Sumner, PhD, Professor, Department Head and Extension Project Leader, Department of Food Science and Technology, Virginia Polytechnic Institute and State University, Blacksburg, Virginia

Liaison from the Board on Health Promotion and Disease Prevention

Hugh Tilson, MD, DrPH, Clinical Professor of Epidemiology and Health Policy and Senior Adviser to the Dean, School of Public Health, University of North Carolina at Chapel Hill

Staff

David A. Butler, PhD, Study Director
Allison Yates, PhD, RD, Director, Food and Nutrition Board
Rose Marie Martinez, ScD, Director, Board on Health Promotion and Disease Prevention
Jennifer A. Cohen, Research Associate
Anna Staton, MPA, Research Assistant
Elizabeth Albrigo, Project Assistant
Rita Gaskins, Division Assistant
Jim Banihashemi, JD, Financial Associate
Melissa French, Financial Associate
Norman Grossblatt, Senior Editor

Staff Consultant

Ricardo Molins, PhD, Senior Staff Officer

Reviewers

This report has been reviewed in draft form by individuals chosen for their diverse perspectives and technical expertise, in accordance with procedures approved by the NRC's Report Review Committee. The purpose of this independent review is to provide candid and critical comments that will assist the institution in making its published report as sound as possible and to ensure that the report meets institutional standards for objectivity, evidence, and responsiveness to the study charge. The review comments and draft manuscript remain confidential to protect the integrity of the deliberative process. We wish to thank the following individuals for their review of this report:

Mindy Brashears, PhD, Texas Tech University
P. Michael Davidson, PhD, University of Tennessee
Colin O. Gill, PhD, Agriculture and Agri-Food Canada
Jimmy T. Keeton, PhD, Texas A&M University
Jørgen Schlundt, DVM, PhD, World Health Organization

Although the reviewers listed above have provided many constructive comments and suggestions, they were not asked to endorse the conclusions or recommendations nor did they see the final draft of the report before its release. The review of this report was overseen by **Stephen L. Taylor**, PhD, University of Nebraska and **Ronald W. Estabrook**, PhD, University of Texas Southwestern Medical Center at Dallas. Appointed by the NRC, they were responsible for making certain that an independent examination of this report was carried out in accordance with institutional procedures and that all review comments were carefully considered. Responsibility for the final content of this report rests entirely with the authoring committee and the institution.

Preface

The efforts of the Committee on the Review of the USDA *E. coli* O157:H7 Farm-to-Table Process Risk Assessment were supported by the work and dedication of the project staff and numerous other individuals who shared their thoughts and expertise with the committee. We could not have completed our task satisfactorily without the substantial help of the these individuals.

We are particularly indebted to Wayne Schlosser and Eric Ebel of the US Department of Agriculture (USDA), who provided detailed information on the draft risk assessment and answered the committee's many questions. Special thanks are also extended to I. Kaye Wachsmuth, Karen Hulebak, Carol Maczka, and Kathleen Orloski of USDA, and Anna Lammerding of Health Canada, for their expert advice and assistance. Edmund Crouch of Cambridge Environmental Inc. contributed a detailed examination of the draft model spreadsheet that is reproduced as Appendix D of this report. Randall Huffman of the American Meat Foundation Institute and Caroline Smith DeWaal of the Center for Science in the Public Interest provided comments for the committee's consideration.

We greatly appreciate the guidance and insights offered by our liaison from IOM's Board on Health Promotion and Disease Prevention, Hugh Tilson. Food and Nutrition Board (FNB) Chair Cutberto Garza, and FNB member Robert Smith provided input on report drafts.

David A. Butler, who served as the study director for this project, worked in concert with Ricardo Molins of FNB to produce this report. The committee would also like to acknowledge the excellent work of IOM staff members Jennifer Cohen, Anna Staton, and Elizabeth Albrigo. Thanks are also extended to Melissa French and Jim Banihashemi, who handled the finances for the project; Norman Grossblatt who provided editorial input; William McLeod, who conducted database searches; Jennifer Otten, who supervised the report through the editorial and publication phases; Bronwyn Schrecker, who shepherded the report through the review process; and Rita Gaskins, who provided administrative support to the project.

Michael P. Doyle, *Chair*

Contents

EXECUTIVE SUMMARY   1
Background, 1
Organization and Framework, 3
Comments Regarding the Draft Risk Assessment, 4

1 SUMMARY OF THE FOOD SAFETY AND INSPECTION SERVICE DRAFT RISK ASSESSMENT   13
Production Module, 14
Slaughter Module, 17
Preparation Module, 22
Hazard Characterization Module, 25
Risk Characterization Module, 26

2 PRODUCTION MODULE   27
Fecal Prevalence as the Sole Output of the Production Module, 28
Defensibility of Prevalence Estimations for Cull Cows and Feedlot Animals, 30

3 SLAUGHTER MODULE   41
Lack of Data and Difficulties Associated with Data Collection, 42
Sources of Contamination and Cross Contamination During Slaughter and Fabrication, 44
Levels and Extent of Surface-Area Contamination, 50
Terminology Concerns, 55
Other Observations, 56
Summary Remarks, 58

4 PREPARATION MODULE 62
Cross Contamination, 62
Modeling in the Preparation Module, 65

5 HAZARD CHARACTERIZATION 71
Review of the Hazard Characterization Chapter, 72
Summary Remarks, 84

6 RISK CHARACTERIZATION 89
Definition of Key Terms, 89
Risk of Illness from *E. Coli* O157:H7, 91
Population Risk by Season, Age, and Location, 94
Sensitivity Analysis, 95
Conclusions, 95
General Comments, 96

7 MODELING APPROACH AND IMPLEMENTATION 97
Description of the Overall Modeling Approach, 98
Description of Model-Updating (Anchoring) Algorithms, 103
Model Validation, 108
Modeling Issues in Hazard Characterization, 109
Software Implementation, 115
Justification of Modeling Assumptions, 121
Overall Model Uncertainty and Reliability, 126

APPENDIXES

A AGENDAS OF PUBLIC MEETINGS HELD BY THE COMMITEE ON THE REVIEW OF THE USDA *E. COLI* O157:H7 FARM–TO–TABLE RISK ASSESSMENT 135

B ADDITIONAL COMMENTS 137

C COMMITTEE AND STAFF BIOGRAPHIES 141

D *E. COLI* ASSESSMENT: SOME COMMENTS BY EDMUND CROUCH, PhD, CAMBRIDGE ENVIRONMENTAL INC. 147

Executive Summary

BACKGROUND

While the US food supply is widely considered to be among the safest in the world, foodborne diseases are still thought to cause some 76 million illnesses, 325,000 hospitalizations, and 5,000 deaths in the country each year (Mead et al., 1999). A 2001 analysis by the US Department of Agriculture (USDA) estimated the annual medical costs, productivity losses, and value of premature deaths due to exposure to five common foodborne pathogens[1] at $6.9 billion (ERS, 2001).

In the face of such a major public health problem, USDA's Food Safety and Inspection Service (FSIS) is formulating risk assessments to identify important foodborne hazards; evaluate potential strategies to prevent, reduce, or eliminate those hazards; assess the effects of different mitigation strategies; and identify research needs. These risk assessments, in brief, empirically characterize the determinants of the presence or level of microbial contamination in vulnerable foodstuffs at various points leading up to consumption.

One of the initial efforts in the undertaking is a risk assessment of the public health impact of *E. coli* O157:H7 in ground beef (USDA-FSIS, 2001).[2] A draft report describing this work was released for comment on

---

[1] The five pathogens are *Campylobacter*, nontyphoidal *Salmonella*, *Escherichia coli* O157:H7, *E. coli* non-O157:H7 STEC, and *Listeria monocytogenes*.

[2] The complete text of the draft risk assessment may be found on the FSIS web site (www.fsis.usda.gov). At the time this report was completed, the URL for the draft was http://www.fsis.usda.gov/OPPDE/rdad/FRPubs/00-023N/00-023NReport.pdf.

September 7, 2001. In addition to soliciting public input, FSIS asked the Institute of Medicine (IOM) to convene a committee of experts to review the draft and offer recommendations and suggestions for consideration as the agency finalizes the document. This report presents the results of that review.

E. coli O157:H7

E. coli serotype O157:H7 is a rare variety of E. coli, a normal inhabitant of the intestines of all animals, including humans (FDA, 2002). The pathogen produces large quantities of one or more related potent toxins, called Shiga toxins, that cause severe damage to the lining of the intestine and to other target organs, such as the kidneys. E. coli O157:H7 was first recognized as a cause of illness in 1982 during an outbreak of severe bloody diarrhea that was later traced to contaminated hamburgers (CDC, 1982). It has since been implicated in a number of outbreaks of intestinal distress. The most severe outcome in the general population is typically hemorrhagic colitis, a prominent symptom of which is bloody diarrhea. Life-threatening complications, however, sometimes ensue. Some victims, particularly the very young, may develop hemolytic uremic syndrome (HUS). HUS, which is characterized by renal failure and hemolytic anemia, occurs in up to 15% of hemorrhagic colitis victims and can lead to permanent loss of kidney function. In the elderly, the combination of HUS with fever and neurologic dysfunction is characteristic of thrombotic thrombocytopenic purpura (TTP). Left untreated, TTP has a mortality of about 95%; however, early diagnosis and treatment yield a survival rate of 80–90% (Abumuhor and Kearns, 2002). Overall, the Centers for Disease Control and Prevention estimates that E. coli O157:H7 is responsible for some 73,500 cases of infection, 2,150 hospitalizations, and 61 deaths in the United States each year (Mead et al., 1999).

Eating meat, particularly ground beef, that has not been cooked sufficiently to kill E. coli O157:H7 is thought to be the primary cause of infection. Cross contamination—which occurs when harmful bacteria in raw beef or its juices are spread to other foods through contact with cutting boards, utensils, and the like—also accounts for illnesses. Among other known sources of infection are consumption of contaminated sprouts, lettuce, salami, and unpasteurized milk and fruit juice; swimming in or drinking contaminated water; and contact with the stools of infected animals or people. FSIS has classified E. coli O157:H7 as an adulterant in raw ground beef, thus banning the sale of any ground beef contaminated with it.[3]

---

[3] Under the Federal Meat Inspection Act, meat is adulterated if it bears or contains any poisonous or deleterious substance, which might render it injurious to health. E. coli O157:H7 has been classified as an adulterant in raw ground beef since 1994.

The Food Safety and Inspection Service

FSIS is the public health agency in the USDA. It is responsible for ensuring that the nation's commercial supply of meat, poultry, and egg products is safe, wholesome, and correctly labeled and packaged.

On July 25, 1996, FSIS issued its landmark rule, *Pathogen Reduction; Hazard Analysis and Critical Control Point (HACCP) Systems* (USDA-FSIS, 1996). The rule addresses foodborne illness associated with meat and poultry products by focusing more attention on the prevention and reduction of microbial pathogens on raw products that can cause illness. FSIS is formulating microbial risk assessments to help to inform efficient risk-management policy decisions and identify future research needs.

The application of risk assessment techniques to microbial pathogens poses challenges that differ from those of chemical, environmental, or toxicologic risk assessments. Notably, bacterial populations are living things that can grow, spread, or die, depending on the characteristics of their environment. FSIS is working with other agencies and institutions to develop appropriate quantitative risk assessment methods and to support studies to fill data gaps and enhance the precision and reduce the uncertainty in risk characterizations of microbial pathogens.

Charge to the Committee

USDA asked the IOM committee to provide comments on the draft *E. coli* O157:H7 risk assessment for consideration as they finalized the document. The charge directed the committee to include evaluations of the overarching logical structure of the model, the validity and appropriateness of the input data used, the reasonableness of the assumptions made, the reasonableness of the anchoring approach (that is, the adjustment of simulation outputs of the model to be more compatible with observed data), and the model's mathematics and equations. It also asked the committee to consider whether risks had been appropriately characterized and whether key sources of variability and uncertainty, critical assumptions, and important data gaps had been identified and characterized.

ORGANIZATION AND FRAMEWORK

The format of this report follows, in part, the organization of the FSIS draft risk assessment. The major topics addressed are

- a summary of the content of the draft risk assessment (Chapter 1);
- reviews of the three modules of the exposure assessment—Production, Slaughter, and Preparation—that characterize the nature and deter-

minants of *E. coli* O157:H7 contamination from the prevalence of the pathogen in cattle on the farm to its presence in a serving of cooked ground beef (Chapters 2–4);

- a review of the Hazard Characterization, the section of the assessment that relates exposure to the pathogen to various health outcomes (Chapter 5); and
- an examination of the Risk Characterization, the part of the assessment that uses the model to generate risk estimates and provides a means for examining which steps in the process are most influential in determining the model's outputs (Chapter 6).

The committee's comments on the overall approach taken for constructing and implementing the model appear in Chapter 7. The FSIS draft also includes a chapter ("Hazard Identification") that summarizes the microbiologic and epidemiologic evidence used in the analysis. The committee's comments regarding this content are in the reviews of later chapters where it is referred to.

An appendix to the report contains an independent review by Edmund Crouch—presented to the committee at a public meeting in February 2002—that provides additional comments on the model's variables and the software implementation of the analysis.

COMMENTS REGARDING THE DRAFT RISK ASSESSMENT

The committee conducted a thorough, science-based examination of the content of the draft—mindful of the fact that it was a work-in-progress—and generated a number of comments focused on the subjects delineated in the charge. Because the report contains specific observations on numerous individual components of a complex assessment, it is not possible to cogently and concisely list all of the comments here. The sections below are a synopsis of the committee's major findings. Chapters 2–7 detail the reasoning underlying these conclusions and present the committee's complete findings.

At the outset, it should be said that the effort underlying the FSIS draft risk assessment is impressive. The authors of the report have undertaken an extraordinary task of collection, analysis, and integration of information that far exceeds the scope and breadth of prior assessments of *E. coli* O157:H7. They faced a number of substantial methodologic hurdles peculiar to microbial risk assessment whose solutions have not been described in textbooks or published elsewhere. It is thus appropriate that they interrupt their effort to allow for peer review and to reassess their solutions to these very challenging issues.

In that regard, the committee commends the draft's authors on the magnitude of their effort and the principles behind it. It wishes to make clear that many criticisms of this model would probably apply to most, if not all, microbial risk assessment efforts previously and currently undertaken.

Production Module

The Production Module of the draft risk assessment models *E. coli* O157:H7 in cows, bulls, steers, and heifers from the farm through transit to the slaughter plant. The committee's principle comment on this section pertains to the use of fecal prevalence as the sole output of the module. It notes that the concentration at which an animal sheds pathogen is also important—one animal shedding 10^5 colony forming units (CFU) of *E. coli* O157:H7/g of feces would yield the same number of cells as 1,000 animals shedding 10^2 CFU/g, yet both are considered to contribute equally in a model in which only prevalence is factored in. The exclusive use of fecal prevalence also requires the assumption that most carcass contamination in later stages of processing occurs directly from the gastrointestinal tract of slaughtered animals, although circumstantial evidence suggests that the hide is also an important source. The decision to use fecal prevalence appears to have been necessitated by the paucity of information on other indicators. The committee thus recommends that the risk assessment acknowledge forthrightly that fecal prevalence is being used as a proxy to characterize several interrelated variables that are poorly understood and on which data are sparse, and that some carcass contamination is derived from contaminated hides. It also recommends that an impact assessment of animals shedding *E. coli* O157:H7 at high and low concentrations be conducted.

The committee raises some questions regarding whether data from disparate studies have been properly combined and whether prevalence has been correctly calculated in all cases, notably in the determination of within-herd prevalence. These instances, detailed in Chapter 2, can be addressed by more clearly defining the intent of the variables estimated in the module and changing the inputs and variable equations as appropriate.

Slaughter Module

The Slaughter Module estimates the prevalence of *E. coli* O157:H7 at each step of the slaughter-plant process, starting with live cattle entering the plant and ending with packaged meat product that is ready for shipment. The committee's primary comments regarding this module also have to do with the lack of available information. The draft risk assessment correctly notes that published data on the prevalence and cell density of *E. coli* O157:H7 during the slaughter and fabrication processes are scarce. In addition, data on the surface area contaminated and the extent of cross contamination are lacking.

The draft recognizes the need for more research to obtain additional information on the contribution of the hide to carcass contamination; the prevalence, extent, and density of *E. coli* O157:H7 contamination on carcasses after dehiding; the contribution of cross contamination to product contamination; the effect of carcass decontamination and chilling on increases or decreases in *E. coli* O157:H7 organisms; and the influence of fabrication activities on redistribution of contamination in meat cuts and trimmings.

The committee observes that the lack of publicly available data regarding crucial steps in the slaughter process, the variability of the operations modeled in the module, and the potential unpredictability of the effects of some activities on contamination during slaughter and carcass fabrication complicate modeling and limit the module's forecasting capacity. The draft module relies heavily on the results of only one study (Elder et al., 2000), makes major assumptions regarding some variables, and readjusts some inputs to fit the expected outcomes. Although such practices are often necessary in model development, the committee recommends that these difficulties and deficiencies be more strongly emphasized in discussions of the outcomes calculated by the model and that the need for more data for model improvement be highlighted throughout the final assessment. Furthermore, the committee recommends that the final assessment stress the potential influence of slaughter plant activities on cross contamination, on the level of contamination, and on the extent of carcass or trim surface area contaminated. It should make clear that the effects of these activities, although important, might be difficult to characterize empirically. The committee recommends that the authors add a discussion of the appropriate and inappropriate applications of the Slaughter Module in its present state of development—in particular, whether the module is ready to be used to draw conclusions about which factors modeled in it are most important in influencing the occurrence and extent of *E. coli* O157:H7 contamination in ground beef and the possible effects of interventions.

Preparation Module

The Preparation Module estimates the incidence and scope of *E. coli* O157:H7 contamination in a serving of cooked ground beef by modeling the conditions under which it is ground, transported, stored, handled, and cooked. A central issue for the committee in its review of this module is the lack of factoring of the contributing influence of cross contamination on human illness. Cross contamination during preparation results when *E. coli* O157:H7 is transmitted from contaminated ground beef to such vehicles as other foods, food preparation and processing surfaces, and food handlers. Because of the highly infectious nature of the pathogen, vehicles cross-contaminated through direct or indirect exposure are likely to be important sources of human illness.

The draft clearly notes that exposures from cross contamination are outside the scope of the assessment, and the committee understands and respects the decision of the modelers to establish reasonable bounds on the reach of their work—a necessary part of any risk assessment. The committee observes, however, that cross contamination during preparation is an established, important risk factor; that the lack of data concerning its impact is no more severe than the lack of data for some other parts of the draft model; and that further attention to cross contamination will help to lay the groundwork for an analysis and better identify the data gaps that need to be filled by future research. The value of the risk assessment in informing public health policy and supporting regulatory interventions will be increased if it is able to factor in the effect of cross contamination on *E. coli* O157:H7 infections and perhaps address the influence of interventions. Just as important, the committee is concerned that the draft risk assessment may foster the incorrect impression that proper cooking of ground beef will prevent all *E. coli* O157:H7 infections associated with ground beef. If the model is used to simulate the impact of various interventions on human health outcomes, the omission of cross contamination could unintentionally omit from consideration interventions that could have a material effect on infection.

The committee thus suggests that consideration be given to factoring cross contamination in the model. If that is not possible, it recommends that the final risk assessment more clearly highlight the role of cross contamination in *E. coli* O157:H7 infection and emphasize the limitations in the model engendered by a decision to not factor it.

The committee notes that although practices for storage, handling, and cooking of ground beef in the home, at fast-food restaurants, and in other retail facilities (called HRI—hotels, restaurants, and institutions—in the draft) vary considerably, the model does not differentiate among them. It suggests that the revised model account for these differences and model each location separately.

Data availability is an issue in this module, as elsewhere. In the draft's calculations of the annual number of raw ground-beef servings, some estimates are unsound because a very small number of observations are linearly extrapolated to represent the entire population. The committee recommends that the authors acknowledge that they do not have adequate information on the consumption of raw ground beef and suggests that alternatives that reflect the uncertainty in the numbers be pursued while better data are sought.

Hazard Characterization Modules

The draft's Hazard Characterization Module describes a method to estimate the number of symptomatic infections resulting from the consumption of cooked ground beef contaminated with *E. coli* O157:H7. As it is not possible to test this relationship directly, upper and lower boundaries for it are established by using data from similar pathogens. Overall, the committee believes that the draft chapter's authors did an elegant job in generating a dose-response function. The available literature strongly supports the relevance of their decision to use data on *Shigella dysenteriae* 1 for the upper limit of the bracket. The data further argue, though, that the *E. coli* O157:H7 dose-response function is likely to be very close to that of *Shigella* and that arguably it will be more appropriate to use dose-response data from experimental challenges with *Shigella* administered with buffer. The use of enteropathogenic *E. coli* (EPEC) dose-response data as the lower limit is reasonable but somewhat more problematic because studies of its effects in humans do not generally reflect real-world exposures. The committee believes that the EPEC dose-response function is a conservative choice and suggests that if the bounding approach is used in the final risk assessment, consideration should be given to alternatives that might reflect *E. coli* O157:H7 pathogenicity better.

More generally, although the draft's discussions of the baseline number of *E. coli* O157:H7 infections and adjustments for underdiagnosis and underreporting are scientifically sound, they do not account for non-O157:H7 serotypes of enterohemorrhagic *E. coli* (EHEC). The virulence properties that allow O157:H7 to cause hemorrhagic colitis, HUS, and TTP are common to a broader category of pathogens. The draft indicates that because *E. coli* O157:H7 is the most important serotype in the United States from a public health standpoint and because there is a paucity of epidemiologic data on non-O157 serotypes, the risk assessment is limited to *E. coli* O157:H7. The committee acknowledges that decision but points out its implication: whatever risk to the public health of the United States is attributed to O157:H7 as a ground-beef contaminant by the risk assessment will be an underestimate of the overall risk because other EHEC serotypes also cause disease. Because non-O157:H7 serotypes contribute to the EHEC disease burden—particularly as a cause of HUS—the committee suggests that the decision to exclude these serotypes be revisited. If the final risk assessment is limited to O157:H7, the committee recommends that this decision and its implications for the model be explicitly discussed in the "Hazard Characterization" chapter.

Risk Characterization

The draft's risk characterization integrates and applies the modeling work done in the three exposure assessment modules (Production, Slaughter, and Preparation) and the dose-response assessment presented in the "Hazard Characterization" chapter to generate analyses of the risk associated with *E. coli* O157:H7 exposure for individuals, the community, and the US population. It is premature to draw conclusions regarding the results of these analyses, because the model is in draft form, but the committee does have some suggestions regarding the form and focus of this work when the model is final.

In particular, the committee believes that the draft's focus on a "typical" individual is—from a public health and policy perspective—misguided. It is desirable to avoid all *E. coli* O157:H7 infections, but attention needs to be centered on the more severe outcomes of infection. The committee therefore recommends that the risk characterization be refocused to concentrate on the analysis of severe illnesses associated with *E. coli* O157:H7 infection, the subpopulations known or thought to be most vulnerable to them, and the interventions that might have the greatest impact on preventing them.

The committee questions the informativeness of the risk estimates generated with the model as it is now structured because it is already adjusted to conform to observed levels of illness. It suggests that a discussion of potential applications of the model's various outputs would be a useful addition to the final assessment. The authors should make clear what they believe the model can and cannot be used for and should address how the structure of the model affects whether particular applications or inferences are appropriate.

Modeling Approach and Implementation

Two major issues were identified in the committee's overall review of how the draft model was constructed and implemented.

The first is that the risk assessment is not structured in the form classically used in such work. A risk assessment is typically an effort directed at providing an estimate of risk through the collection of evidence and the application of mathematical tools, and the risk estimate is usually a dependent output of the model. The draft alters that arrangement by deriving the exposure assessment and the population risk estimates from separate sources and then inferring an *E. coli* O157:H7 dose-response relationship that is mathematically compatible with the calculated exposure assessment and the distribution of population risk estimates.

The committee recommends that the final report more clearly communicate the nature of, the rationale for, and the impact of the deviation from the standard approach and that the authors consider relabeling the product as a *system risk model* to avoid implying that the model generates an estimate of risk independent of those derived from epidemiologic estimates. It also recommends that the authors re-evaluate the approach taken to infer the dose-response relationship in light of the possibility that this parameter is not the greatest source of uncertainty in the model and in consideration of other comments expressed in this review.

At several points in the development of the draft model, algorithms are invoked to adjust the simulation outputs to be more compatible with observed data. That technique, called *anchoring* in the report, is well-founded in health risk assessment and the related field of environmental modeling. But its use poses three problems that the committee believes should be more completely addressed. First, by censoring some simulation outcomes, valuable information on low-probability adverse events may be lost. Second, the rationale underlying the choice and management of censored values is not well articulated. Third, the ability to validate the model through comparison with observed events or the output of other *E. coli* O157:H7 risk assessments is compromised. The authors should consider removing the current algorithms for calculating dose-response parameters and replacing them with model elements based on evidence that is independent of O157:H7 epidemiologic data. That will allow for a stable evidence base and provide for some limited validation of model estimates with epidemiologic data. If no independent data are available, a formal statistically based updating algorithm could be used.

The other major issue is the transparency with which the draft model is presented—the extent to which "the rationale, the logic of development, constraints, assumptions, value judgements, decisions, limitations and uncertainties of the expressed determination are fully and systematically stated, documented, and accessible for review" (Codex Alimentarius Commission, 1999). Appendix C to the draft (released as a supplement on October 9, 2001)—a partial list of the model equations and code—is a good start in this effort. However, as noted in several instances in the committee's review, the final assessment needs to make explicit the major assumptions underlying the model. Details of all the variables and equations used must be clearly listed, including data sources, units of measure, and distribution shapes as appropriate. And the analysis environment (now a spreadsheet with macros to automate the simulation process, implemented with and without "add-in" software to generate some statistical distributions) needs to be documented in a fashion that allows other professionals to more easily track the flow of the equations and trace errors. The credibility of the risk assessment will be greatly enhanced if its structure and inner workings are made more clearly visible to the outside world.

The management of uncertainty (a deficiency in the knowledge base) and variability (the dispersion or distribution of some known quantity) is a challenge in all risk assessments. The committee's review notes specific instances in which a thorough effort to characterize quantities by, for example, reconstructing regression scatters or modeling sampling error of empirical distributions would be appropriate.

A somewhat related question is the management of intervariable dependences. The draft treats all variables in a given equation as uncorrelated with one another. That assumption makes implementation of simulations more straightforward but does so at the possible expense of precision. The committee suggests that the authors evaluate available empirical information related to possible correlations among the variables and, in the absence of relevant data, carefully consider whether independence assumptions are most appropriate for the model.

General Comments

Two unifying concepts underlie many of the committee's comments on the draft risk assessment. Both are universal in the field of risk assessment. The first concept is that the risk assessment will be improved by making the inner workings of the analysis more explicit so that others may understand it better. Model building is a complex process, and the more accessible it is to others, the better the opportunities for its use and improvement. The second is that the lack of data on major components of the process being modeled hampers the construction of an informative risk assessment. Risk assessments are intended to collect and format knowledge in a way that is useful to decision-makers. Identification of data gaps is thus a strength of the process. The data deficiencies identified in the FSIS risk assessment should serve as the foundation for a delineation of research priorities to be promoted or pursued so that the model and *E. coli* O157:H7 policy decisions can be improved in the future.

REFERENCES

Abumuhor I, Kearns EH. 2002. Thrombotic Thrombocytopenic Purpura. The Virtual Health Care Team, School of Health Professions and the School of Medicine, University of Missouri, Columbia. www.vhct.org/case2300/morbidity.shtml, accessed March 14, 2002.

CDC (Centers for Disease Control). 1982. Epidemiologic Notes and Reports: Isolation of *E. coli* O157:H7 from Sporadic Cases of Hemorrhagic Colitis—United States. Morbidity and Mortality Weekly Report 31(43):580, 585.

Codex Alimentarius Commission. 1999. Principles and Guidelines for the Conduct of Microbiological Risk Assessment. CAC/GL-30. Food and Agricultural Organization of the United Nations.

Elder RO, Keen JE, Siragusa GR, Barkocy-Gallagher GA, Koohmaraie M, Laegreid WW. 2000. Correlation of enterohemorrhagic *Escherichia coli* O157 prevalence in feces, hides, and carcasses of beef cattle during processing. Proceedings of the National Academy of Sciences 97(7):2999–3003.

ERS (Economic Research Service), US Department of Agriculture. 2001. ERS Estimates Foodborne Disease Costs at $6.9 Billion per Year. www.ers.usda.gov/Emphases/SafeFood/features.htm, accessed July 30, 2002.

FDA (Food and Drug Administration) 2002. *Escherichia coli* O157:H7. Center for Food Safety & Applied Nutrition Foodborne Pathogenic Microorganisms and Natural Toxins Handbook. vm.cfsan.fda.gov/~mow/chap15.html, accessed March 14, 2002.

Mead PS, Slutsker L, Dietz V, McCaig LF, Bresee JS, Shapiro C, Griffin PM, Tauxe RV.1999. Food-related illness and death in the United States. Emerging Infectious Disease 5(5):607–625.

USDA-FSIS (US Department of Agriculture, Food Safety and Inspection Service). 1996. Pathogen Reduction; Hazard Analysis and Critical Control Point (HACCP) Systems; Final Rule. Part II, 9 CFR Part 304, et al. Federal Register: July 25, 1996 61(144):38805–38956.

USDA-FSIS. 2001. Draft Risk Assessment of the Public Health Impact of *Escherichia coli* O157:H7 in ground beef. September 7, 2001. [Draft report Appendix C dated October 9, 2001; Appendix D undated but released October 31, 2001.]

1

Summary of the Food Safety and Inspection Service Draft Risk Assessment

The stated purpose of the draft risk assessment prepared by the Food Safety and Inspection Service (FSIS) of the US Department of Agriculture (USDA) is to systematically evaluate and integrate available scientific data and information to

- provide a comprehensive evaluation of the risk of illness from *E. coli* O157:H7 in ground beef based on currently available data,
- estimate the likelihood of human morbidity and mortality associated with specific numbers of *E. coli* O157:H7 in ground beef servings,
- estimate the occurrence and extent of *E. coli* O157:H7 contamination at points along the farm-to-table continuum,
- provide a tool for analyzing how to most effectively mitigate the risk of illness from *E. coli* O157:H7 in ground beef,
- identify future food safety research needs, and
- assist FSIS in the review and refinement of its integrated risk reduction strategy for *E. coli* O157:H7 in ground beef (p. 1).[1]

The attendant model follows each step of the production process, from the prevalence of the pathogen in cattle on the farm to its presence in a single serving of cooked ground beef.

---

[1] The complete text of the draft risk assessment may be found on the FSIS web site (www.fsis.usda.gov). At the time this report was completed, the URL for the draft was www.fsis.usda.gov/OPPDE/rdad/FRPubs/00-023N/00-023NReport.pdf.

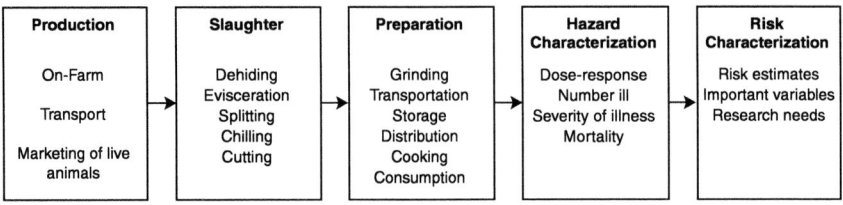

FIGURE 1-1 Risk-assessment structure for *E. coli* O157:H7 in ground beef. (Reproduced from USDA-FSIS (2001) Figure 1-1.)

This chapter summarizes the content of the FSIS risk assessment as presented in the draft report and is intended as a reference for readers who do not have ready access to that document.[2] The draft risk assessment itself is reviewed in the next five chapters and the modeling approach and implementation in Chapter 7.

The model is divided into three exposure assessment modules (Production, Slaughter, and Preparation), a Hazard Characterization Module (also known as dose-response assessment), and a Risk Characterization Module, which estimates the risk of illness from *E. coli* O157:H7 in ground beef. Figure 1-1 is a graphic representation of those components, which are discussed below.

PRODUCTION MODULE

The Production Module estimates the prevalence of *E. coli* O157:H7 in live cattle entering US slaughter plants. *Prevalence*, in this context, is the proportion of a population that is infected. In the model, cattle are divided into two groups: breeding cattle (mature cattle bred to produce milk and calves) and feedlot cattle (steers and heifers specifically intended for slaughter). The distinction is made because breeding and feedlot cattle differ in their slaughter and in the processing and distribution of their meat, and because some evidence suggests that *E. coli* prevalence varies between the two groups of cattle. About 20% of all cattle slaughtered in the United States are breeding cattle; the remaining 80% are feedlot cattle. Some 15% of beef consumed in the United States is imported from other countries; the model assumes that any *E. coli* O157:H7 contamination in imported beef would be equivalent to that in domestic beef.

---

[2] References for the statements made in the chapter are listed in the draft report.

The Production Module is divided into three segments: on-farm, transportation, and marketing of live animals (referred to as slaughter-plant intake in the FSIS draft risk assessment). Those segments, discussed below, represent the three phases that all breeding and feedlot cattle go through before slaughter.

On-Farm Segment

The primary focus of the on-farm segment in the FSIS model is to evaluate the prevalence of *E. coli* O157:H7 in herds of cattle on the farm before they are sent to slaughter. Cattle are often tested on the farm to determine whether *E. coli* O157:H7 is present in herds. Fecal testing is used to find *infected* cattle—cattle whose intestinal tracts are colonized with the *E. coli* O157:H7 organism. Cattle that test positive for O157:H7 on their hides, hair, or hooves are labeled as *contaminated*.

Prevalence can be evaluated in a herd in many ways. The four critical inputs to the Production Module are *herd prevalence* and *within-herd prevalence* of *E. coli* O157:H7 for both breeding and feedlot cattle. Herd prevalence is the proportion of herds of a particular type (breeding or feedlot) that have at least one *E. coli* O157:H7-infected animal; it is assumed to remain constant at a national level. Within-herd prevalence is the proportion of *E. coli* O157:H7-infected animals in an infected herd.

Another variable considered in the on-farm segment of the FSIS model is seasonal variability, the tendency for *E. coli* O157:H7 prevalence in a herd to increase or decrease with the time of the year. Evidence suggests that there is a high-prevalence season (June to September) and a low-prevalence season (October to May). That is important because increasing the proportion of cattle entering the slaughter process that test positive for *E. coli* O157:H7 could lead to an increase in its prevalence in ground beef.

Data for the on-farm segment of the model were collected from published research articles that contained information about the prevalence of *E. coli* O157:H7 in herds on farms throughout the United States. The data were evaluated to estimate the mean and 5th and 95th percentiles of *E. coli* O157:H7 prevalence. The estimates consistently showed that *E. coli* O157:H7 prevalence is significantly higher in feedlot cattle than in breeding cattle. An evaluation of herd prevalence and within-herd prevalence in breeding and feedlot cattle did not alter that finding. The findings were consistent whether or not seasonality was considered.

Transportation Segment

The transportation segment considers the transmission of *E. coli*

O157:H7 among cattle being shipped from the farm to the slaughter plant. There is a potential for *E. coli* O157:H7 to be transmitted from infected to uninfected cattle or for animals that tested positive for *E. coli* O157:H7 on the farm to lose the infection en route. Research has not shown any marked increase or decrease in the fecal prevalence of *E. coli* O157:H7 among cattle that are first tested on the farm before transport and then retested at the slaughter plant. There are no data that document *E. coli* O157:H7 prevalence on cattle hides at the farm and after transport to slaughter. For those reasons, no effect of transport is included in the model.

Slaughter Plant Intake Segment

All breeding and feedlot cattle are transported to a slaughter plant from livestock markets or farms by trucks. Because breeding cattle are not specifically raised for slaughter, it is not uncommon for them to make their way to livestock markets and then slaughter plants individually rather than in an established herd from one farm. Therefore, it is assumed that the prevalence of *E. coli* O157:H7 among breeding cattle is independent of that in other cattle that may arrive at the same time. Only in the unlikely event that a large group of breeding cattle (over 40 cows) arrive at a slaughter plant from one farm at the same time would that not be the case.

To model the prevalence of infected breeding cattle in each truckload arriving for slaughter, a Monte Carlo simulation is used. In a Monte Carlo simulation, random values are generated for uncertain variables over and over again to simulate myriad possible outcomes. In the FSIS model, the Monte Carlo simulation is generated from the expected number of cattle (40) in each truckload, herd prevalence, and within-herd prevalence. The technique is also used to evaluate the effect of low- and high-prevalence seasons on the pervasiveness of *E. coli* O157:H7.

Slaughter-plant intake of feedlot cattle varies from that of breeding cattle. Feedlot cattle are generally transported directly from their original feedlot to the slaughter plant and slaughtered together as a group. Because each truckload of feedlot cattle originate from the same pen in a feedlot, all the cattle on board have the same probability of being infected with *E. coli* O157:H7. A separate Monte Carlo simulation is generated for feedlot cattle under the assumption that each truckload of cattle originates from an infected or non-infected feedlot based on feedlot prevalence and seasonality.

The inputs generated from these simulations, which provide a prevalence distribution for the number of infected cattle entering the slaughter plant, are used as the starting numbers (inputs) for the Slaughter Module.

SLAUGHTER MODULE

The Slaughter Module estimates the prevalence of *E. coli* O157:H7 at each step of the slaughter-plant process, starting with live cattle entering the plant and ending with packaged meat product that is ready for shipment. Breeding and feedlot cattle are modeled separately. High- and low-prevalence seasons, representing the times of year when cattle are slaughtered, are also modeled separately. Only cattle that are slaughtered and processed in commercial plants are considered in the model.

Many factors influence whether *E. coli* O157:H7 will end up in the final meat product. Even if cattle begin the slaughter process infected or contaminated with *E. coli* O157:H7, it will not always be found in the meat after processing. Contamination or decontamination can occur at any step of the slaughter process. Therefore, one must take many other factors into account when evaluating the presence of *E. coli* O157:H7 during the slaughter process, including the status of the cattle entering the slaughter plant, the type of processing plant, the type of equipment used and procedures followed within the plant, and the efficiency of the decontamination and sanitation processes.

In the model, the slaughter process is divided into seven steps: the arrival of cattle at the slaughter plant, dehiding, decontamination after dehiding (first decontamination), evisceration, second decontamination, chilling, and carcass fabrication. Those steps are detailed below.

Arrival of Live Animals

Cattle arrive at slaughter plants by truck from farms and livestock markets. After arrival, they are placed in holding pens at the plant until they are led to slaughter. The model does not provide any information about the level of *E. coli* O157:H7 transmission that occurs in the holding pens at the plants. The estimated prevalence of *E. coli* O157:H7 in each truckload of arriving cattle—calculated in the Production Module by the type of cattle and the season—serves as the initial set of inputs for the Slaughter Module.

The model estimates the prevalence of *E. coli* O157:H7 in processed meat after slaughter on the basis of prevalence in each truckload of cattle arriving at the plant. To determine the amount of processed meat that will come from each truckload of cattle, some assumptions are made. For each truckload of cattle, a total carcass weight is estimated. The carcass weight is the weight of an animal after it has been killed and its hide has been removed. Average carcass weights have been determined for each type of cattle: breeding cattle (dairy cattle and calves) and feedlot cattle (steers and heifers). Summing the average carcass weights based on the distribution of cattle in each truckload results in a total carcass weight per truckload. The average truckload is assumed to be 40 cattle.

Once the carcass weight has been estimated, further calculations are used to establish how much of the carcass will be processed as distinct cuts of meat and how much will be trim, the meat product from which ground beef is eventually made. Trim is made up primarily of muscle and fat; it is the remainder after the cuts of meat have been removed from feedlot cattle. In breeding cattle, trim is the primary product after deboning of the carcass. Trim is removed from each carcass and combined into 2,000-pound combo bins during the slaughter process. Combo bins are typically large cardboard boxes lined with plastic that are used to collect meat trim. The percentage of each carcass that amounts to trim is calculated as a percentage of the total carcass weight for each cattle type. The number of live cattle necessary to fill one combo bin is called a *lot* in the FSIS draft report.

To summarize, the goal in this first step of the Slaughter Module is to estimate the number of trucks per lot. That is calculated by using the type of cattle in the truckload to determine the average carcass weight and the amount of trim from each carcass. From those data, the number of animals needed to fill one combo bin (one lot) is determined on the basis of a truckload of 40 cattle. By using the final outputs of the Production Module as the inputs in the Slaughter Module, the prevalence of *E. coli* O157:H7 in each lot can now be determined on the basis of calculations from each truckload of cattle entering the slaughter plant.

Knock Box and Stunning (Not Modeled)

Cattle entering the slaughter plant are channeled into the "knock box," where they are stunned. After stunning, the animals are chained to an overhead conveyer rail by one hind leg. Before moving on the conveyer to the main floor of the slaughter plant, an animal's throat is slit and the animal is bled. Although cross-contamination can occur during this part of the slaughter process, it is not included in the model, because data on hide contamination, the most likely contamination in this part of the slaughter process, are lacking.

Dehiding

In the next step of the process, the animal is moved to the main floor of the slaughter plant, and the dehiding process begins. To remove the hide from the animal, thus creating a carcass, the horns, hocks (joints of leg to foot), and udder are removed. The head is skinned and the hide is cut down the midline, legs, and front shanks and rolled up over the carcass.

There are many opportunities for contamination to occur during the dehiding process. If the hide is intact before dehiding, E. coli O157:H7 contamination is limited to the surface of the hide and the feces. Once the hide is removed, the sterile muscle and fat on the carcass are exposed to microbial contamination. Contamination of the carcass can occur directly from its own hide or feces (self-contamination); from other infected carcasses via clothing, gloves, knives, or machinery in the plant; and through the release of aerosols from contaminated carcasses during the dehiding process.

To evaluate contamination during the dehiding process, a *transformation ratio* is created; it is defined as the ratio of the frequency of contaminated carcasses to the frequency of infected cattle in a lot (as determined in the "Arrival of Live Animals" step). The prevalence of E. coli O157:H7 on carcasses is calculated from data contained in a paper by Elder and colleagues (2000), which are used to estimate the range of carcass contamination during the high-prevalence season. To estimate the lower frequency of contamination during the low-prevalence season, the same data are used, but more uncertainty is introduced into the calculation by creating a "mixture" of the transformation ratio and a uniform distribution, which ranges from near zero to a maximum of the transformation ratio found during the high season.

On the basis of data from research papers and the FSIS national baseline survey of slaughter plants (1994), further calculations are made to estimate the maximum and minimum number of E. coli O157:H7 organisms on a contaminated carcass at dehiding. The results of the calculations provide the basis of modeling the next step of the slaughter process.

First Decontamination

To remove any visible foreign matter after dehiding, one or more decontamination processes may be used to clean the carcass. Large areas of fecal contamination, defined as those greater than 1 inch in diameter, are removed with a knife. Smaller areas of contamination are removed by spot steam vacuuming. Some plants decontaminate the entire carcass with a hot-water rinse or organic acids. No procedure is successful in removing all E. coli O157:H7. Visible contamination can be reduced from the carcass surface with knives and vacuuming, but some bacterial colonies—invisible to the naked eye—will be missed. In addition, cross-contamination from improperly cleaned knives, clothing, and equipment can occur during the decontamination process. Using rinsing during the decontamination process will reduce the E. coli O157:H7 on the carcass but might not remove all the contamination. To account for any residual contamination after the first decontamination process, the model factors in a variable to represent the reduction of *E. coli* O157:H7 on the carcass. Three reduction values are represented in the model in a triangular distribution—a minimum, an uncertain "most-likely" value, and an uncertain maximum—to capture the various levels of decontamination success.

Evisceration

In the evisceration step, the carcass is split along the ventral midline, and the gastrointestinal tract and remaining organs (including bladder, lungs, and heart) are removed. Although opportunities for contamination are slight at this stage, it can occur if the intestinal tract is perforated during removal and there is leakage onto the surrounding muscle tissue. The model presumes that if the animal is already infected with *E. coli* O157:H7 and leakage occurs during evisceration, contamination will occur.

Carcass Splitting (Not Modeled)

During carcass splitting, the carcass is sawed in half, the tail is removed, and excess fat is trimmed away from the sides. Although it is possible for contamination to occur during these procedures, it has not been modeled because there are no relevant data available.

Second Decontamination

The first and second decontamination steps are similar in that knives and spot steam vacuuming are used to remove visible contamination from carcasses. The model assumes that small plants use, in addition, hot-water rinsing, sometimes with organic acids. This rinsing can either reduce the *E. coli* O157:H7 on the surface or redistribute it over the entire carcass. The effectiveness of rinsing is assumed to be the same as in the first decontamination. The model also assumes that larger plants typically use steam pasteurization during their second decontamination. Although that can be highly effective in reducing contamination on carcasses, studies have shown that variation in the steam-pasteurization process can affect its efficacy. To model the variation, a minimum, an uncertain most-likely value, and an uncertain maximum are used to represent steam-pasteurization efficacy.

Chilling

After the second decontamination, the split carcasses are placed into a blast air chiller for 24–48 hours. The sides of beef are occasionally sprayed with water or in some cases other solutions. After chilling, the sides are unloaded, graded, and sorted. The model accounts for the possibility of growth of or decline in *E. coli* O157:H7 on the surface of an already-contaminated carcass during the chilling process because of fluctuations in time and temperature. No new contamination is assumed to occur in this step.

Carcass Fabrication

After carcasses are removed from the chiller, they move on overhead rails to the fabrication floor for cutting and deboning. In plants that slaughter feedlot cattle, major and minor (primal and subprimal) cuts of meat are removed from the carcass by slaughter plant personnel with knives. "Leftover" trim, primarily muscle and fat, is separated and collected. Breeding cattle are processed in the same way, but trim is a primary product rather than a byproduct that results from deboning. Once the trim is removed from the carcass, it moves on conveyer belts to combo bins or to vacuum-packaging areas. Trim going to combo bins is packed with dry ice in preparation for shipping. The remainder of the trim is vacuum-packed, packaged in boxes, and chilled at 0°–2°C (32.0°–35.6°F) until shipping.

Although few studies have looked exclusively at contamination that occurs during carcass fabrication, there are many opportunities for *E. coli* O157:H7 contamination and cross-contamination. Not only can contamination take place as trim from different animals is combined in combo bins, but it can also come from contact with processing and cutting equipment and from workers' gloves and aprons. And although fabrication areas are kept at a temperature intended to inhibit growth (10°C, or 50°F), higher temperatures can occur that will lead to increases in the growth of *E. coli* O157:H7.

The model estimates the level of contamination that occurs during fabrication by creating a simulation using the outcomes from the slaughter process and the grinder segment of the Preparation Module (which uses FSIS sampling data). High- and low-prevalence seasons are factored in separately. The model anchors the output of this section to real-world observations by placing bounds on how the generated values are used: if simulation results are too high, they are discarded; if they are too low, contamination is added in the model to reflect contamination during fabrication. Results from this portion of the model indicate that the fabrication process is critical with respect to *E. coli* O157:H7 contamination.

Slaughter Module Results

The final outputs of the Slaughter Module—which become the inputs for the Preparation Module—are the distributions of *E. coli* O157:H7 in the trim in combo bins and boxes at slaughter plants. The distributions take into account the type of cattle being slaughtered (feedlot or breeding) and the time of year when the animals are slaughtered (high- and low-prevalence seasons).

The distributions generated by the Slaughter Module suggest that *E. coli* O157:H7 contamination is higher in feedlot cattle than in breeding cattle and that the prevalence and levels of contamination found in combo bins and boxes is greater during the high-prevalence season. The model indicates that an average of 6% and 8% of combo bins produced from breeding cattle are contaminated with one or more *E. coli* O157:H7 organisms during the low and high seasons, respectively; an average of 23% and 43% of combo bins containing meat from feedlot cattle are contaminated during the low- and high-prevalence seasons. The disparity in prevalence between breeding and feedlot cattle is due primarily to variations in their living conditions, feeding practices, and processing before they enter the slaughter plant.

Boxes of processed meat follow the same general pattern of contamination as combo bins. Of boxes generated from breeding cattle, 1–2% are contaminated with at least one *E. coli* O157:H7 organism during the low and high seasons, respectively. Within boxes of meat trim from feedlot cattle, an average of 6% and 13% are contaminated during the low and high seasons. Although the averages are lower for boxes than for combo bins, the decreases reflect the fact that boxes contain much less trim than combo bins (60 pounds versus 2,000 pounds) and therefore fewer servings. Overall, the risk of consuming contaminated ground beef processed from boxes and combo bins would be roughly equivalent.

PREPARATION MODULE

The Preparation Module estimates the incidence and scope of *E. coli* O157:H7 contamination in a single serving of cooked ground beef. For the model, *ground beef* is defined as hamburger patties or formed major ingredients (such as meatballs or meatloaf). Factors examined include handling practices and cooking, the age of the consumer, and the location where the ground beef is cooked. Cross-contamination is considered to be beyond the scope of the model and is therefore not included.

The Preparation Module is divided into six steps: grinding beef trim, storage during processing by the retailer or distributor, transportation to the home or to a large-scale establishment (termed an HRI for hotels, restaurants, and institutions), storage at home or "away from home", cooking, and consumption (whose evaluation takes into account the age of the consumer and the location of the meal).

Grinding Beef Trim

As described earlier, the outputs of the Slaughter Module serve as the inputs for the grinding step of the Preparation Module. Those outputs are the distributions of *E. coli* O157:H7 in the trim that fills the combo bins and boxes at slaughter plants (taking into account cattle type and season). Each combo bin has a level of "leanness" that is defined by the fat in the animals that contributed to the trim. To produce ground beef with a specific fat content, it is necessary to combine trim from different combo bins. Trim from breeding cattle is routinely mixed with trim from feedlot cattle. In the United States, 60% of trim comes from feedlot cattle (steers and heifers); the remainder comes from breeding cattle (cows and bulls). About 15% of all beef consumed in the United States is imported. Imported beef is either processed separately or mixed with domestic product. The model assumes that contamination in imported meat is equivalent to that in domestic meat.

Trim from combo bins is processed in large commercial facilities. The model combines combo bins of three types of beef trim (from domestic breeding and feedlot cattle and from imported cattle) to represent the mixing that occurs during the grinding process. Grinder loads are presumed to vary in size from the equivalent of 2 to 15 combo bins of trim. If there is any *E. coli* O157:H7 contamination in a bin before grinding, it is assumed to be distributed throughout the load during grinding. A further calculation is made for retail ground meat that is modeled as coming from one to seven 60-pound boxes of trim.

Once ground beef is processed, it is sold by wholesale distributors to retail establishments (grocery stores, butcher shops, and the like) and HRI that in turn sell it to consumers. Retail operations buy ground beef in "case-ready chubs" (plastic tubes filled with 5–10 pounds of ground beef) and use it directly or mix the processed ground beef with trim produced in house. Generally, HRI use ground beef directly as it comes from grinder establishments.

Storage by Retailer or Distributor, Transportation to Home or HRI, and Storage at Home or "Away from Home"

The next part of the FSIS draft model examines *E. coli* O157:H7 contamination in beef from the time it is ground until the time it is ready to be prepared for consumption. Various factors can affect how much *E. coli* O157:H7 growth, if any, occurs during this time: the storage time and temperature (including effects of freezing), the fat content, the strain of *E. coli* O157:H7, and the packaging.

To model growth of *E. coli* O157:H7 in ground beef, three assumptions are made.

- All areas of a product are at the same temperature.
- All *E. coli* O157:H7 strains exhibit the same growth characteristics in any ground-beef product.
- The lag period (the time before cell division) in any stage is affected by temperatures in previous stages.

Information on the time between purchase and cooking and on storage temperatures is used to predict microbial growth or inhibition.

Cooking

The cooking portion of the Preparation Module simulates the effect of cooking on *E. coli* O157:H7 in ground beef in homes and HRI. The model uses data from a survey of final internal temperatures of cooked product. To determine the effect of cooking on *E. coli* O157:H7, the model simulates the internal cooking temperature and variables that represent pretreatment storage conditions (time and temperature of storage). Differences in hamburger patty thickness are not explicitly modeled.

Consumption

Three primary types of ground beef are modeled in the consumption portion of the Preparation Module: raw ground beef, hamburger patties and sandwiches, and such products as meatballs and meatloaf whose major ingredient is formed ground beef. Consumption patterns at and away from home and the age of the consumer are factored in. Data for this modeling come from the USDA's 1994–1996 and 1998 Continuing Survey of Food Intakes by Individuals (CSFII) (Kause, 2001). To calculate the amount of ground beef consumed, the model factors in the three ground-beef options above and uses survey data that indicate the frequency with which meals are consumed at and away from home. That results in two eating locations and three meal options—a total of six possible combinations for ground-beef consumption. The amount of ground beef in each ground-beef food item is modeled by using CSFII's recipe files. The model further stratifies the data into four age categories (0–5, 6–24, 25–64, and 65+ years). Of primary interest are the youngest and oldest consumers (0–5 and 65+ years) because these groups are the most susceptible to the ill effects of *E. coli* O157:H7 contamination.

HAZARD CHARACTERIZATION MODULE

The Hazard Characterization Module seeks to characterize the dose-response relationship for *E. coli* O157:H7, that is, how the amount of pathogen consumed affects the risk of infection, illness, or death. In this context, a *dose* is the number of *E. coli* O157:H7 organisms in a serving of ground beef. The *response* refers not only to the number of people who get ill from consuming *E. coli* O157:H7-contaminated ground beef but also to the severity of illnesses. Because *E. coli* O157:H7 infection has the potential to induce serious illness and cause death, it is not possible to conduct dose-response testing on human subjects; the model must rely on information accumulated from other sources to make the calculations in this module.

To determine how many cases of *E. coli* O157:H7-induced illness occur in the United States annually, information was gathered from the 1996–1999 Emerging Infections Program, Foodborne Disease Active Surveillance Network (FoodNet). Dose-response estimates are calculated by using the FoodNet data and input from the exposure-assessment modules regarding amounts of *E. coli* O157:H7 in servings of cooked ground beef. Adjustments are made to account for underreporting and overreporting of infections in the FoodNet data and to ensure that the *E. coli* O157:H7 dose-response estimates are consistent with those known for other pathogens. Further calculations are used to estimate the number of severe cases of illness from *E. coli* O157:H7 infection that will result in hospitalization or death and to determine which age groups are most susceptible to infection.

To set the upper and lower boundaries of the *E. coli* O157:H7 dose-response function, data from similar ("surrogate") pathogens were used. After evaluation of the availability of data, genetic relatedness, and similarities in transmission, infectivity, and pathogenicity, *Shigella dysenteriae* 1 was chosen as the upper-boundary pathogen. That is, it was assumed that exposure to a given dose of *E. coli* O157:H7 was no more capable of causing illness than exposure to an equivalent dose of *Shigella dysenteriae* 1. Enteropathogenic *E. coli* (EPEC) was chosen as the lower-boundary pathogen.

A dose-response function for *E. coli* O157:H7 is then derived by using the upper- and lower-boundary dose-response functions in conjunction with the estimated number of cases attributed to ground beef and the estimated number of servings contaminated with *E. coli* O157:H7. Dose and response information from an outbreak of *E. coli* O157:H7 due to contaminated ground beef is then compared with the derived function to "validate" it (that is, demonstrate that it generated results consistent with an actual event).

RISK CHARACTERIZATION MODULE

The Risk Characterization Module of the FSIS draft model estimates the risk and severity of illness from the consumption of a single serving of *E. coli* O157:H7-contaminated ground beef. They are calculated for different populations (from individuals to entire communities), exposures (single, per year, or during a lifetime), and population variability (season, age, and where the meal was prepared). To make those estimates, the model combines outputs from the Exposure Assessment and Hazard Characterization modules.

A risk characterization can be used to help to identify the steps in a process that have the greatest influence on the final output and thus highlight where interventions may be most effective. When the risk assessment is final, such analyses will assist FSIS in the review and refinement of its integrated risk-reduction strategy for *E. coli* O157:H7 in ground beef.

REFERENCE

Elder RO, Keen JE, Siragusa GR, Barkocy-Gallagher GA, Koohmaraie M, Laegreid WW. 2000. Correlation of enterohemorrhagic *Escherichia coli* O157 prevalence in feces, hides, and carcasses of beef cattle during processing. Proceedings of the National Academy of Sciences 97(7):2999–3003.

FSIS (Food Safety and Inspection Service). 1994. Nationwide Beef Microbiological Baseline Data Collection Program: Steers and heifers—October, 1992–September, 1993.

Kause J. 2001. SAS Analysis of the 1994–1996, 1998 CSFII for Consumption of Ground Beef by Age and Location for the *E. coli* O157:H7 Risk Assessment. Informational memorandum to Wayne Schlosser through Carol Maczka, Director, Risk Assessment Branch, Office of Public Health and Sciences, Food Safety and Inspection Service, USDA, Washington, DC.

USDA-FSIS (US Department of Agriculture, Food Safety and Inspection Service). 2001. Draft Risk Assessment of the Public Health Impact of *Escherichia coli* O157:H7 in Ground Beef. September 7, 2001. [Draft report Appendix C dated October 9, 2001; Appendix D undated but released October 31, 2001.]

2

Production Module

The purpose of the Production Module is to estimate the prevalence of *E. coli* O157:H7-infected cattle entering US slaughter plants. The justification is that the prevalence of *E. coli* O157:H7 in slaughter cattle influences its occurrence on carcasses and ultimately in ground beef. At least three studies lend empirical support to the premise that infected cattle are a direct source of carcass contamination. Bonardi et al. (2001) and Chapman et al. (1993) reported an association between fecal positivity and carcass positivity at the level of the individual animal or carcass. Elder and colleagues (2000) found a correlation between combined fecal and hide prevalence of *E. coli* O157:H7 in groups of cattle (slaughter lots) and the prevalence on carcasses. An analysis of pulse-field gel electrophoresis profile isolates from the study by Elder et al. (2000) found high concordance between fecal and carcass isolates within slaughter lots (Barkocy-Gallagher et al., 2001). The common seasonal pattern, in temperate climates, of *E. coli* O157:H7 fecal prevalence in cattle (Hancock et al., 1997a; Heuvelink et al., 1998), retail meats (Chapman et al., 2001), and humans (Wallace et al., 2000) also lends credibility.

The utility of the estimates of fecal prevalence from the Production Module depends on the answers to two central questions that are discussed in detail below.

- Is fecal prevalence alone an adequate measure of output for the Production Module?
- Are the prevalence estimates in cull cows (called "breeding cattle"

in the Fod safety and Inspecton Service (FSIS) draft risk assessment) and feedlot animals defensible?

FECAL PREVALENCE AS THE SOLE OUTPUT OF THE PRODUCTION MODULE

The arguments against using fecal prevalence alone for risk assessment are related to the wide range of concentrations of E. coli O157:H7 in the feces of colonized cattle and the fact that E. coli O157:H7 occurs in locations other than feces.

On theoretical grounds, animals shedding 10^5 colony-forming units (CFU) of E. coli O157:H7 per gram of feces would cause much more contamination of meat than animals shedding, say, 10^2 CFU/g, but they are considered to contribute equally in a model that includes only prevalence. The issue might not be of concern if the distribution of pathogen concentrations were narrow or if one could assume a dependable relationship, at the group level, between prevalence and distribution of concentrations. However, the distribution clearly is not narrow. Experimentally infected animals often reach peak shedding concentrations over 10^5 CFU/g briefly and typically shed much lower numbers for longer periods (Cray and Moon, 1995; Sanderson et al., 1999). Some cattle that are naturally exposed to an infected animal never shed over 10^3 CFU/g (Besser et al., 2001). There is a paucity of data on shedding dynamics in field populations, but the seeming consequence of findings from challenge studies is that one would expect only a small fraction of positive animals in a group to be shedding E. coli O157:H7 at over 10^5 CFU/g on any given day. However, those few animals probably account for the large majority of total E. coli O157:H7 cells produced by the group. The disjunction between prevalence and quantity of E. coli O157:H7 shed has probably been magnified as tests have become more sensitive because, as documented by Sanderson et al. (1995) and Besser et al. (2001), the major impact of increased sensitivity of an assay is its ability to detect lower concentrations. For example, methods based on immunomagnetic separation (IMS) have allowed far better detection of animals shedding 10^2 CFU/g than older assays (Besser et al., 2001). But one animal shedding 10^5 CFU/g would yield the same number of E. coli O157:H7 cells as 1,000 animals shedding 10^2 CFU/g.

The use of fecal prevalence as the sole output of the Production Module requires the assumption that most carcass contamination with E. coli O157:H7 (or fecal bacteria in general) occurs directly from the gastrointestinal tracts of slaughtered animals. The draft defends that assumption by reference to a study showing little or no correlation between visible hide soiling and generic E. coli counts on carcasses (Van Donkersgoed et al.,

1997) and several studies suggesting that hide prevalence is lower than fecal prevalence. Admittedly, it is difficult to find studies that provide quantitative data on the source of bacteria contaminating carcasses, but circumstantial evidence suggests that the hide is a major source of carcass contamination (Castillo et al., 1998; Midgley and Desmarchelier, 2001). Visible soiling of hides and carcass contamination may correlate poorly because of the failure to distinguish between visible and microbiological hide soiling. That is, it may be that the level of microbiological contamination cannot be judged visually. The lower prevalence on hides than in feces may be due to the sampling of only a tiny fraction of the hide in the cited studies or to the lower sensitivity of IMS expected for an environmental sample. Only 450 cm^2 of the hide was sampled, and sorbitol-negative bacteria resistant to cefixime and tellurite are more common in hide than in fecal samples and can interfere with identification of *E. coli* O157:H7. Moreover, although Elder et al. (2000) found 28% fecal prevalence versus 11% hide prevalence, the carcass prevalence was reported to be 43.4%. It seems unlikely that such a large percentage of carcasses were contaminated with feces directly from the rectum or with other gastrointestinal contents.

The use of fecal prevalence of *E. coli* O157:H7 as the output of the Production Module without consideration of the concentration of *E. coli* O157:H7 in feces or contamination of hides and hooves was seemingly necessitated by the paucity of data on anything beyond fecal prevalence. It appears that fecal prevalence is thus being used as a proxy variable to define several interrelated variables that are poorly understood and on which data are scarce. That is not an insurmountable problem, especially given the aforementioned studies demonstrating a correlation between fecal prevalence and carcass contamination. Use of fecal prevalence of *E. coli* O157:H7 alone does allow at least a crude assessment of the effect of farm-level interventions on the extent of ground-beef contamination, but it is possible to imagine that an intervention might reduce concentration, especially at the high end, and have little or no effect on prevalence. For example, if the reduction in prevalence resulted in fewer animals shedding 10^3 CFU/g or less but did not impact the prevalence of animals shedding >10^3, then the overall impact on amount of total number of *E. coli* O157:H7 cells shed by a group of animals would be negligible. Also, important sites for intervention, such as transport and confinement conditions or methods of hide removal, may be excluded from the draft risk assessment if fecal prevalence is the sole output of the Production Module. The exclusion of effects of preslaughter transport and lairage from the model may need re-examination in light of a report of increasing *E. coli* O157:H7 prevalence with increasing number of transit points (Cornell Collaborative Project, 1998). Although only a small minority of cattle had multiple transit points, such uncommon occurrences may have a substantial effect on *E. coli* O157:H7 contamination of ground beef. Furthermore, a paper by Midgley and Desmarchelier (2001) documents the occurrence of a subtype of *E. coli* O157:H7 (and also shigatoxic O26:H11) on hides of animals sampled at slaughter that had never been observed on intensive sampling during the feeding period of these animals; this suggests that the subtype had been acquired during confinement at the slaughter plant. Although the sample size evaluated by Midgely and Desmarchelier was too small to allow a judgment of the quantitative impact of lairage, more recent papers by Small et al. (2002) and Avery et al. (2002) suggest that the lairage effect might be substantial. On the other hand, another recent paper (Barham et al., 2002) reported a significant decline in prevalence from the feedlot to the slaughter plant.

For those reasons, the committee recommends that the final risk assessment acknowledge forthrightly that fecal prevalence is being used as a proxy variable and that some carcass contamination is derived from hides.

DEFENSIBILITY OF PREVALENCE ESTIMATES FOR CULL COWS AND FEEDLOT ANIMALS

Pooling data from disparate studies that had differing assay methods and sampling designs is difficult, and the draft risk assessment does a generally credible job. However, several issues related to adjustment for imperfect sensitivity of tests and to estimation of within-herd prevalence, herd prevalence, and seasonal effects merit scrutiny.

Issues Related to Adjustment for Test Imperfections

Possible Specificity Problems

Theoretically, errors of two kinds can be made by a test: false negatives (imperfect sensitivity) and false positives (imperfect specificity). The draft risk assessment rightly devotes considerable attention to false negatives in its discussion of test sensitivity, but the potential for false positives is not raised. The most likely reasons for false positives are the incorrect identification of *E. coli* O157:H7 and cross contamination. While the former is not an evident problem in any of the studies cited, the latter is a potential problem, especially in studies that use IMS. Cross contamination of IMS samples is a problem that is to be expected in the absence of specific controls (PHLS, 2000). The two key issues for avoiding false positives are the use of blank tubes in each run and the capping of all tubes except the one tube being immediately processed (PHLS, 2000). Unless the authors of a paper state (or, if asked, can state) that those procedures were adhered to and that blanks were uniformly negative, it must be assumed that false positives probably occurred. In any case, it seems unreasonable to go to considerable lengths to address imperfect test sensitivity while failing to note the possibility of imperfect test specificity. **The committee suggests that the final risk assessment note that imperfect specificity was not assessed but may have had an impact on the output of the Production Module.**

Estimating Prevalence of E. coli O157:H7 in Feces Requires Specification of Target Detection Limit

In contrast with the apparent assumption of Table 3-4 in the FSIS draft risk assessment, no procedure is capable of detecting one *E. coli* O157:H7 organism in a sample. As shown by Sanderson et al. (1995), every *E. coli* O157:H7 assay procedure has a 50% detection end point—the concentration at which half the positives are detected and half are missed—that is substantially greater than one organism per sample (or per gram). Every procedure (including IMS, in contrast with the draft risk assessment's assumption of 100% sensitivity) has false negatives, even for occasional samples with concentrations of several powers of 10 above the 50% detection end point. It is also clear that as one collects more volume of feces and performs more replicate tests, the probability of detecting *E. coli* O157:H7 increases asymptotically in a fashion that has no obvious end point short of one cell per daily fecal output. If one organism per daily fecal output is considered an absurd boundary separating positive from negative results, one is left to define the reasonable boundary. Any such attempt will confront unresolvable arguments of whether it is colonization, infection, or simple shedding (including passive) that one wants to measure and whether a level of fecal shedding can even separate these states. The lack of any reasonable gold standard for *E. coli* O157:H7 fecal testing and the seemingly unfathomable problem of selecting an end point fecal concentration combine to make a convincing case for using the concentration of fecal shedding of *E. coli* O157:H7, rather than simple prevalence, as an output of the Production Module. That is so because the increasing numbers of animals shedding asymptotically lower levels of *E. coli* O157:H7 contribute little to the overall amount of *E. coli* O157:H7 shed into the environment (and ultimately onto carcasses). If one accounts for animals shedding *E. coli* O157:H7 at over 10^3 CFU/g, one has surely accounted for over 99% of total *E. coli* O157:H7 shedding. Although data on the concentration of fecal *E. coli* O157:H7 shedding are sparse, they should be sufficient to allow estimation of the relative effect of high-level shedders (say, over 10^4 CFU/g) compared with low-level shedders. **The committee recommends that the risk assessment provide an impact assessment of animals shedding *E. coli* O157:H7 at high and low levels.** The committee notes that there is a paucity of information on this topic[1] and suggests that the risk assessment highlight the need for more research.

Issues Related to Computation of Within-Herd Prevalence

Data from Juvenile Cattle May Have Been Included

Two of the within-herd prevalence estimates in Table 3-2 of the FSIS draft included juvenile animals (Besser et al., 1997; Hancock et al., 1994), whereas the intent was to estimate prevalence in adult animals. It is possible that only data from adults were extracted from the studies to obtain the tabulated values; if so, this should be made clear. The data on the distribution of within-herd prevalence shown in Figure 3-3 of the draft were collected exclusively from juvenile animals and should not be used to estimate the distribution of within-herd prevalence in adult animals; a number of studies have shown a higher prevalence of *E. coli* O157:H7 in juvenile than in adult cattle (Hancock et al., 1997a; Heuvelink et al., 1998). However, it is acceptable (even desirable) to include data on juveniles in determining herd prevalence, as was done in draft's Table 3-1. **The committee recommends that the risk assessment not use data on juvenile animals to estimate within-herd prevalence in adult animals.**

Distribution of Within-Herd Prevalence Ignores Temporal Clustering Effect

Within a herd, the prevalence of *E. coli* O157:H7 seems to be unevenly distributed in time; bursts of prevalence occur periodically (Hancock et al., 1997a; Sargeant et al., 2000). Thus, a prevalence study in which each farm is sampled on a single occasion or a small number of occasions would be expected to find a wide distribution of within-herd prevalence even if long-term within-herd prevalence in the herd was identical. Indeed, a distribution much like those in Figures 3-5 and 3-10 of the FSIS draft risk assessment could be generated from multiple sampling visits to a single herd. Only by pooling data across many herd visits—as was done in the study by Hancock et al. (1997b), on which Figure 3-3 is based—can one obtain a reasonable picture of distribution of within-herd prevalence. However, it could be argued that the goal of risk assessment is best met by estimating the daily distribution of within-

---

[1] A study of the concentration of *E. coli* O157:H7 in the feces of juvenile cattle by Zhao et al. (1995) already cited in the draft is an exception.

herd prevalence (because cull cows are shipped on particular days rather than on average days). If that argument is accepted, a distribution based on pooling of multiple sampling visits, such as that portrayed in Figure 3-3, should not be used. **The committee recommends that a decision be made as to whether distribution of within-herd prevalence by herd-day *or* by herd is more appropriate for the model and that only studies relevant to the chosen metric be used.**

Estimates Are Biased by Use of Within-Herd Prevalence Data Only in Positive Herds

Use of data only on herds *detected* as positive (in contrast with herds *actually* positive), especially if samples per herd are relatively small, results in a biased estimate of within-herd prevalence and its distribution. The effect is most evident in studies with very small samples. If, for example, only five samples were collected per herd in a large number of herds, the herds detected as positive would be estimated to have a minimum of 20% prevalence even if the true within-herd prevalence were 1%. Although no studies with a within-herd sample size of five were included in Table 3-2 in the draft, the effect exists even with larger samples. It is evident in considering the extremely high estimates from Hancock et al. (1994) shown in Table 3-5 in the FSIS draft risk assessment (the estimate in Table 3-2 adjusted for sensitivity). If a very insensitive culture method was used, the sample size of 60 per herd in the Hancock et al. paper was not adequate to detect positive herds reliably. That expectation was confirmed by a follow-up study in which four of eight herds initially found to be negative were later found to be positive after more-intensive sampling (Hancock et al., 1997a). An accurate estimate of within-herd prevalence cannot be reasonably made from small samples unless one makes a priori assumptions about herd prevalence. That is, the denominator of the within-herd prevalence estimate would need to include not only the number of sampled animals from herds that were detected as positive, but also those from herds that were truly positive but, because of inadequate sample size, were not detected as positive. Practically speaking, that cannot be done unless one assumes 100% herd prevalence, which, on the basis of intensive sampling studies, is probably closer to reality than what has been depicted in the draft risk assessment. **The committee recommends that the FSIS draft risk assessment either compute within-herd prevalence estimates as the total positives divided by the total sampled (herd status notwithstanding) or use a denominator based on the estimated herd prevalence, such as that depicted in Figure 3-2 of the draft.**

Stage on Feed Was Not Considered for Feedlot Data

The largest study thus far published on *E. coli* O157:H7 in feedlot cattle (Hancock et al., 1997c) found a prevalence about three times higher in early-on-feed cattle (those that have recently entered the feed lot) than in late-on-feed cattle (those that will soon be slaughtered). In multivariate modeling of the data (Dargatz et al., 1997), the effect was found to exist in all regions sampled and for two independent sets of data assayed at two laboratories. If the goal is to estimate prevalence in slaughter cattle (late-on-feed), it is inadvisable to include data from cattle at all stages on feed. **The committee recommends that the modelers adjust the estimate for prevalence in feedlot animals to that expected for preslaughter (late-on-feed) animals.**

Prevalence Data on All Adults in Herd Might Not Yield a Good Estimate of Cows Soon to Be Culled

At least two studies (Garber et al., 1999; Rice et al., 1997) have reported higher prevalence in dairy cows identified for culling (but still on the farm) than in adult herdmates. Hence, the use of the within-herd prevalence in all adults may yield a biased estimate of prevalence of cull dairy cattle at the time of slaughter. **The committee suggests that the risk assessment note as a possible weakness that prevalence estimates in cull cattle might be higher than those in all adult cattle.**

Issues Related to Computation of Herd Prevalence

Elder et al. Data on Slaughter Lots Were Used Inappropriately

Data from Elder et al. (2000) were used in computing herd-prevalence in feedlots (Table 3-6 in the draft). The study did not sample individual feedlots, but rather slaughter lots—groups of 35–85 animals from a single source presented for slaughter on a particular day. It is not clear that all 29 of such lots sampled were from independent sources (that is, from 29 separate feedlots). If the Elder et al. data are derived from a relatively small number of separate feedlots, then the calculation of feedlot (herd) prevalence and the assumption that the sample is representative of feedlots in general become problematic. Beyond these simple mathematical issues lies a larger one that raises concerns regarding Elder and colleagues' use of post exsanguination samples from slaughter lots to estimate feedlot prevalence. The committee identifies two questions for the consideration of the modelers:

- Can one accurately determine if a feedlot is positive or negative for *E. coli* O157:H7 by taking a highly clustered sample of a relatively small number of the cattle in a feedlot?

- Can one accurately make this estimate from a set of samples collected after exsanguination and hence after contact with pens and equipment of a slaughter plant that have been reported to be an important source of *E. coli* O157:H7 contamination (Avery et al., 2002; Small et al., 2002)?

The committee recommends that the risk assessment use only data from independent feedlots to estimate herd prevalence in feedlots.

Herd-Prevalence Estimates Erroneously Assume Homogeneous Prevalence over Time in Positive Herds

Computation of the herd-level sensitivity (Equation 3.3 in the draft) and thus herd prevalence appears to depend on an assumption of homogeneous within-herd prevalence. The strong temporal clustering observed for *E. coli* O157:H7 in a herd (Hancock et al., 1997a; Sargeant et al., 2000) invalidates the use of the equation. Consider that a herd with an average within-herd prevalence of, say, 5% will often, on any random sampling occasion, have much less than this prevalence and will occasionally have a much higher prevalence. In a study that uses only one or a few sampling points per herd, one will intercept many of the herds at a within-herd prevalence much below the long-term average, hence invalidating computations like those in Equation 3.3 (which is more appropriate for relatively stable measures, such as seroprevalence). The issue becomes more critical if some of the sampling visits are in winter, when underlying prevalence is lower (Hancock et al., 1994). It is worth noting that the lowest estimate of herd prevalence in the draft's Table 3-4 was derived from the study with the fewest sampling points ($N = 1$ to 3; Garber et al., 1999) whereas studies that used more sampling visits per herd found much higher herd prevalences. Stated differently, the distribution of uncertainty in breeding-herd prevalence (Figure 3-2 in the draft risk assessment) was biased downward by use of an inappropriate means of computing herd sensitivity. The problem is more serious when one considers the feedlot data summarized in Table 3-6 in the draft, where the two studies reporting less than 100% herd prevalence involved only one sampling point per feedlot (Dargatz et al., 1997; Elder et al., 2000). On a theoretical basis it is difficult to imagine how any feedlot that receives cattle and feeds from many sources would not be at least intermittently positive for *E. coli* O157:H7. Inasmuch as the data in Table 3-6 are consistent with 100% herd prevalence in feedlots, one should probably use 100% as the estimate. In

Bayesian terms, there are good a priori reasons to believe that the herd prevalence in feedlots would be 100%, and, unless the data were inconsistent with this, 100% should be used. It is even possible to invoke this argument for breeding herds, but the lower incoming animal traffic and the failure, in some herds, to find any *E. coli* O157:H7 after collecting hundreds of samples at many times suggest that some small percentage of breeding herds remain free of *E. coli* O157:H7 over long periods.

The committee recommends that the risk assessment use an appropriate means of adjusting for herd sensitivity that incorporates effects of temporal clustering for breeding herds *or* base the estimate of herd prevalence only on studies in which breeding herds were sampled multiple times. For feedlots, the committee recommends that a 100% herd prevalence be used.

Issues Related to Estimation of Seasonal Effects on Prevalence

There are good reasons to provide a seasonal adjustment of the prevalence output from the Production Module. First, *E. coli* O157:H7-associated disease in humans is strongly seasonal (Wallace et al., 2000), and at least one study has attributed this to seasonal variation in prevalence of *E. coli* O157:H7 in retail beef and lamb meat (Chapman et al., 2001). Several longitudinal studies in dairy farms and feedlots have provided evidence of a marked seasonal effect (Hancock et al., 1997a; Heuvelink et al., 1998; Mechie et al., 1997; NAHMS, 2001), and some point-sampling studies corroborate it (Bonardi et al., 2001; Hancock et al., 1994; Van Donkersgoed et al., 1999). However, the seasonal prevalences estimated in the draft risk assessment are not the best ones possible.

Two technical mistakes were made in the data depicted in Table 3-5 in the draft:

- Besser et al. (1997) was erroneously used instead of the companion paper, Hancock et al. (1997a). Since the former did not examine seasonal effect, the weighted averages are erroneously displayed as an adjusted 4.5% prevalence throughout the year (presumably on the assumption that if season was not mentioned there must not have been a seasonal effect). In Hancock et al. (1997a)—the companion paper on the same herds in which the effect was examined—a strong seasonal effect was reported.

- In two of the studies (Hancock, 2001; Sargeant et al., 2000), the monthly estimates do not appear to have been adjusted for test sensitivity, although these adjustments were made in other studies.

Beyond those technical mistakes, the methods by which evidence from various longitudinal and point-prevalence studies were combined merit close scrutiny. The problem is most evident in the handling of data from Hancock et al. (1994). In that study, 60 dairy herds were sampled one time each, but sampling was distributed roughly equally in each of the 12 calendar months—that is, about 300 animals in five herds were sampled in each calendar month. But no data (numerator *or* denominator) were included in Table 3-5 from herds or months in which positives were not found, presumably on the assumption that one would never observe a herd prevalence of zero on a sampling visit (say, in winter) to a truly positive herd. That assumption is not valid, as shown by Hancock et al. (1997a) and Sargeant et al. (2000). In both those studies, *most* sampling visits to positive herds were associated with completely negative results. If data from point-sampling studies (such as Garber et al., 1999; Hancock et al., 1994; Rice et al., 1997) are to be used in computing seasonal effect, the only reasonable way to treat them is as generally random surveys of the cattle population (ignoring herd, because herd status cannot be assessed accurately in such studies). Hence, one would not put the same prevalence in each month for point-sampling studies where no clear-cut seasonal effect was found. Rather, one would use the observed prevalence computed as the total positives found divided by the total samples tested, regardless of whether samples came from herds that were, by chance, found to contain positive animals or herds in which no positives were found. It is worth noting that when the data in Hancock et al. (1994) are treated in this manner, a seasonal effect is observed that is similar to that found in a year-long longitudinal study of a subset of the same herds (Hancock et al., 1997a).

Another possible approach that is worth considering is to separate the estimation of prevalence from the estimation of seasonal effect completely. A seasonal adjustment (multiplier) would be made to prevalence estimates from various studies in a manner similar to that for the adjustments for test sensitivity. That would allow one to restrict the computation of seasonal adjustment factors to longitudinal studies done over a year's period—that is, the ones that are most appropriate to the unbiased estimation of seasonal effect. It would also potentially allow inclusion of high-quality longitudinal studies from areas outside the United States, such as that by Heuvelink et al. (1998). It is arguable that conditions peculiar to European cattle production might result in differences in overall average prevalence, but it seems more reasonable to assume that the magnitude of seasonal differences would be similar to that experienced by cattle herds in similar climatologic areas of the United States. Given the paucity of longitudinal studies in the United States, especially those using modern detection technology, the use of data from other countries is worth considering in the estimation of seasonal effects.

The committee recommends the following changes for estimating seasonal effects:

- Use data from Hancock et al. (1997a) instead of Besser et al. (1997).
- Adjust all monthly prevalence estimates for imperfect test sensitivity.
- Either handle the data from multiple surveys as random surveys of the cattle population, thus using data on all cattle sampled in each month, or use only data from longitudinal studies to estimate seasonal adjustment factors.

REFERENCES

Avery SM, Small A, Reid CA, Buncic S. 2002. Pulsed-field gel electrophoresis characterization of Shiga toxin-producing *Escherichia coli* O157 from hides of cattle at slaughter. Journal of Food Protection 65(7):1172–1176.

Barham AR, Barham BL, Johnson AK, Allen DM, Blanton JR, Miller MF. 2002. Effects of the transportation of beef cattle from the feedyard to the packing plant on prevalence levels of *Escherichia coli* O157 and *Salmonella* spp. Journal of Food Protection 65(2):280–283.

Barkocy-Gallagher GA, Arthur TM, Siragusa GR, Keen JE, Elder RO, Laegreid WW, Koohmaraie M. 2001. Genotypic analyses of *Escherichia coli* O157:H7 and O157 nonmotile isolates recovered from beef cattle and carcasses at processing plants in the Midwestern states of the United States. Applied Environmental Microbiology 67(9):3810–3818.

Besser TE, Hancock DD, Pritchett LC, McRae EM, Rice DH, Tarr PI. 1997. Duration of detection of fecal excretion of *Escherichia coli* O157:H7 in cattle. Journal of Infectious Diseases 175:726–729.

Besser TE, Richards BL, Rice DH, Hancock DD. 2001. *Escherichia coli* O157:H7 infection of calves: Infectious dose and direct contact transmission. Epidemiology and Infection 127(3):555–560.

Bonardi S, Maggi E, Pizzin G, Morabito S, Caprioli A. 2001. Faecal carriage of verocytotoxin-producing *Escherichia coli* O157 and carcass contamination in cattle at slaughter in northern Italy. International Journal of Food Microbiology 66(1-2):47–53.

Castillo A, Dickson JS, Clayton RP, Lucia LM, Acuff GR. 1998. Chemical dehairing of bovine skin to reduce pathogenic bacteria and bacteria of fecal origin. Journal of Food Protection 61(5):623–625.

Chapman PA, Siddons CA, Wright DJ, Norman P, Fox J, Crick E. 1993. Cattle as a possible source of verocytotoxin-producing *Escherichia coli* O157 infections in man. Epidemiology and Infection 111(3):439–447.

Chapman PA, Cerdan Malo AT, Ellin M, Ashton R, Harkin. 2001. *Escherichia coli* O157 in cattle and sheep at slaughter, on beef and lamb carcasses and in raw beef and lamb products in South Yorkshire, UK. International Journal of Food Microbiology 64(1-2):139–150.

Cornell Collaborative Project. 1998. Prevalence of *E. coli* O157:H7 Pre-slaughter/*E. coli* O157:H7 Associated Risk Factors. New York State Cull Cow Sub-Project. Final report.

Cray WC, Moon HW. 1995. Experimental infection of calves and adult cattle with *E. coli* O157:H7. Applied Environmental Microbiology 61:1586–1590.

Dargatz DA, Wells SJ, Thomas LA, Hancock DD, Garber LP. 1997. Factors associated with the presence of *Escherichia coli* O157 in feces in feedlot cattle. Journal of Food Protection 60:466–470.

Elder, RO, Keen JE, Siragusa GR, Barkocy-Gallagher GA, Koomaraie M, Laegreid WW. 2000. Correlation of enterohemorrhagic *E. coli* O157 prevalence in feces, hides, and carcasses of beef cattle during processing. Proceedings of the National Academy of Sciences 97(7):2999–3003.

Garber L, Wells S, Schroeder-Tucker L, Ferris K. 1999. Factors associated with the shedding of verotoxin-producing *Escherichia coli* O157 on dairy farms. Journal of Food Protection 62(4):307–312.

Hancock DD. 2001. Personal communication. Ongoing research project in collaboration with FDA-CVM.

Hancock DD, Besser TE, Kinsel ML, Tarr PI, Rice DH, Paros MG. 1994. The prevalence of *Escherichia coli* O157 in dairy and beef cattle in Washington State. Epidemiology and Infection 113:199–207.

Hancock DD, Besser TE, Rice DH, Herriott DE, Tarr PI. 1997a. A longitudinal study of *Escherichia coli* O157 in fourteen cattle herds. Epidemiology and Infection 118:193–195.

Hancock DD, Rice DH, Herriot DE, Besser TE, Ebel ED, Carpenter LV. 1997b. Effects of farm manure handling practices on *Escherichia coli* O157 prevalence in cattle. Journal of Food Protection 60(4):363–366.

Hancock DD, Rice DH, Thomas LA, Dargatz DA, Besser TE. 1997c. Epidemiology of *Escherichia coli* O157 in feedlot cattle. Journal of Food Protection 60(5):462–465.

Heuvelink AE, Van den Biggelaar FL, Zwartkruis-Nahuis J, Herbes RG, Huyben R, Nagelkerke N, Melchers WJ, Monnens LA, de Boer E. 1998. Occurrence of verocytotoxin-producing *Escherichia coli* O157 on Dutch dairy farms. Journal of Clinical Microbiology 36(12):3480–3487.

Mechie SC, Chapman PA, Siddons CA. 1997. A fifteen month study of *E. coli* O157:H7 in a dairy herd. Epidemiology and Infection 118(1):17–25.

Midgley J, Desmarchelier P. 2001. Pre-slaughter handling of cattle and Shiga toxin-producing *Escherichia coli* (STEC). Letters in Applied Microbiology 32(5):307–311

NAHMS (National Animal Health Monitoring System). 2001. *Escherichia coli* O157 in United States Feedlots. USDA: Animal and Plant Health Inspection Service Bulletin #N345.1001.

PHLS (Public Health Laboratory Service). 2000. Laboratory cross contamination of *Escherichia coli* O157 in a sample of organic mushrooms. Public Health Laboratory Service (England and Wales), November.

Rice DH, Ebel ED, Hancock DD, Herriott DE, Carpenter LV. 1997. *Escherichia coli* O157 in cull dairy cows on farm and at slaughter. Journal of Food Protection 60(11):1386–1387.

Sanderson MW, Gay JM, Hancock DD, Gray CC, Fox LK, Besser TE. 1995. Sensitivity of bacteriologic culture for detection of *Escherichia coli* O157:H7 in bovine feces. Journal of Clinical Microbiology 33(10):2616–2619.

Sanderson MW, Besser TE, Gay JM, Gay CC, Hancock DD. 1999. Fecal *Escherichia coli* O157:H7 shedding patterns of orally inoculated calves. Veterinary Microbiology 69(3):199–205.

Sargeant JM, Gillespie JR, Oberst RD, Phebus RK, Hyatt DR, Bohra LK, Galland JC. 2000. Results of a longitudinal study of the prevalence of *E. coli* O157:H7 on cow-calf farms. American Journal of Veterinary Research 61(11):1375–1379.

Small A, Reid CA, Avery SM, Karabasil N, Crowley C, Buncic S. 2002. Potential for the spread of *Escherichia coli* O157, *Salmonella*, and *Campylobacter* in the lairage environment at abattoirs. Journal of Food Protection 65(6):931–936.

Van Donkersgoed J, Jericho KWF, Grogan H. 1997. Preslaughter hide status of cattle and the microbiology of carcasses. Journal of Food Protection 60(12):1502–1508.

Van Donkersgoed J, Graham JT, Gannon V. 1999. The prevalence of vertoxins, *E. coli* O157:H7 and *Salmonella* in the feces and rumen of cattle at processing. Canadian Veterinary Journal 40:332–338.

Wallace DJ, Van Gilder T, Shallow S, Fiorentino T, Segler SD, Smith KE, Shiferaw B, Etzel R, Garthright WE, Angulo FJ. 2000. Incidence of foodborne illnesses reported by the foodborne diseases active surveillance network (FoodNet)-1997. Journal of Food Protection 63(6):807–809.

Zhao T, Doyle MP, Shere J, Garber L. 1995. Prevalence of enterohemorrhagic *Escherichia coli* O157:H7 in a survey of dairy herds. Applied and Environmental Microbiology 61(4):1290–1293.

3

Slaughter Module

The Slaughter Module examines how handling practices and fabrication procedures influence *E. coli* O157:H7 contamination from the time when live cattle arrive at a slaughter plant to the time when pieces of trim are combined into boxes or bins destined for commercial ground-beef production. O157:H7 prevalence distributions developed in the Production Module serve as inputs to this module; its outputs are distributions of O157:H7 contamination in combo bins and trim boxes. The model separately factors in breeder and feedlot cattle and high-prevalence (June–September) and low-prevalence (October–May) seasons.

It is important to recognize that the slaughtering and fabrication processes that constitute the Slaughter Module may be the most crucial link, before cooking for consumption, in the farm-to-fork chain. The importance of the Slaughter Module is evident in the fact that through its steps sterile muscle tissue of healthy animals is converted into meat that may become contaminated with bacteria, including *E. coli* O157:H7. Interventions in the Production Module influence the extent (prevalence) and level (concentration of cells) of contamination introduced into the slaughter plant; interventions in the Preparation Module aim at eliminating the pathogen from the product before consumption. The Slaughter Module bridges the two, examining the factors that affect the amount of fecal and hide contamination that is introduced into and remains on carcasses and how this contamination is distributed on the meat cuts and trimmings that become ground beef. The extent and level of contamination in turn influence the efficacy of cooking in eliminating pathogens from the ready-to-eat product and thus human exposure. Excessive contamination levels may lead to consumer illness due to pathogen survival even after recommended cooking procedures, and high prevalence of contamination at lower levels makes illness from undercooking or cross contamination more likely. Thus, the events evaluated in the Slaughter Module greatly influence the outcome of the whole model.

This chapter presents the committee's review of the Slaughter Module. Five primary subjects are addressed: difficulties of data collection, sources of contamination and cross contamination during slaughter and fabrication, the levels (cell density) and extent of carcass and trim surface-area contamination, the effects of decontamination on pathogen prevalence (especially on pathogen load and surface area contaminated), and terminology. Some additional committee observations and comments are offered in Appendix B, and Appendix D is an independent review prepared by Edmund Crouch on the variables used in this module and their implementation in the spreadsheet environment.

LACK OF DATA AND DIFFICULTIES ASSOCIATED WITH DATA COLLECTION

To those unfamiliar with predictive modeling but with some experience in slaughter operations and microbiology, it may be difficult to understand how modeling could be used to predict contamination levels and the size of surfaces contaminated during slaughter and fabrication operations. The task would seem intractable because of the variability and potential unpredictability of events during those operations. Variability in contamination and cross contamination may originate in such factors as plant size, design, age, equipment, automation, speed of slaughter, and animal holding facilities; geographic location; season of the year; type, lot, and origin of animals; labor shift; and personnel training and turnover. As live animals arrive for slaughter, they may be free of *E. coli* O157:H7 contamination or be contaminated in their gastrointestinal systems or on their hides. Contamination may be localized or may have spread to larger or multiple locations of the hide; the concentration of cells in contaminated spots or niches may be variable. Hide contamination is unpredictable because it can be the result of fecal shedding by individual animal or of cross contamination on the farm, during transportation, or holding before slaughter, when animals enter the slaughter chain. Cross contamination can affect other animals or the plant environment, which in turn can contaminate animals, carcasses, or meat. Fed steers and heifers from one pen are shipped and slaughtered together; culled animals from different farm environments can be commingled and thereby contaminate one another.

Slaughter presents numerous opportunities for contamination and cross contamination that may vary among plants. As the hide is separated for removal, contamination may be introduced onto the carcass surface. A single source (an animal or the plant environment and equipment) may contaminate carcasses not only during dehiding but also during later steps. Some operations are more likely than others to result in carcass contamination, and some carcass areas are more prone than others to exposure to potential contamination or cross contamination; but the prevalence (number of carcasses), extent or level (cell density), and size of the carcass surface area contaminated—especially the latter two—are difficult to estimate, or data are unavailable or impossible to collect for their estimation. During slaughter operations, there is always the opportunity for unpredictable cross contamination or spreading, removal, or inactivation of contamination.

Contamination of a carcass, especially with *E. coli* O157:H7, may be localized and of low or high density. The contamination is not always spread uniformly throughout a given area of the carcass surface. When a carcass sample is analyzed and reported to have a number of some kind of cells per square centimeter, those cells may have actually been present in the whole area being measured or in any fraction of it. The presence and extent of contamination and the size of surface area contaminated with the cells may change unpredictably during the slaughtering steps because of such events as carcasses touching each other, aerosols, worker activities, water splashing, knife trimming, steam vacuuming, spray washing, other decontamination interventions, and surface drying during chilling. Changes in contamination may include elimination, spreading to larger carcass surface areas, shifting to other carcass surface areas, direct cross contamination of other carcass areas through equipment or workers, reduction in numbers or in surface area contaminated, and reduction in prevalence. Those uncertainties do not include potential effects and variation due to differences in bacterial attachment and biofilm formation on surfaces, exposure to sublethal stresses, potential development of bacterial cell resistance, and cross-protection effects of such stresses or interventions as cooking (Samelis et al., 2001a,b, 2002a,b). There are no data for estimating or predicting any of those potential changes, and some of them may prove to be unpredictable. Available data exist only to support the suggestion that dehiding results in carcass contamination (in terms of prevalence) and that decontamination interventions can have a substantial effect in reducing prevalence and levels of contamination if applied properly. Considering the limitations of sampling and testing, those conclusions are well established. However, even for such well-established effects, there is variation among plants, lots of animals, slaughter times, and other factors. Thus, it is difficult to predict the extent (cell density) and the carcass surface area contaminated as a carcass leaves the slaughtering room and enters the chiller. The effect of the chiller on levels of contamination is also largely unknown because of the paucity of data. It is feasible to determine its effect with well-designed studies—but not knowing the carcass area contaminated is still a limitation.

After the chiller, carcass sides enter the fabrication process. Again, the only data that are available or could be obtained with reasonable certainty are related to the prevalence of a pathogen on carcass sides (with all the limitations of sampling); the extent of carcass area contaminated and levels of contamination are still unknown and highly unpredictable. The limitation in data becomes more pronounced during fabrication: carcasses are cut into parts; a major portion of the external carcass surface is removed and enters the rendering process; new and larger meat surfaces are exposed to potential contamination; meat comes into contact with table surfaces, equipment, and worker's hands; and meat from different carcasses is mixed in combo bins. Contamination changes during fabrication are unknown and may be unpredictable.

The scientists who prepared the FSIS draft risk assessment have done a commendable job of developing their model, given the challenges they faced. However, the lack of publicly available data on crucial steps in the slaughter process, the variability of the operations modeled in the module, and the potential unpredictability of the effects of some activities on contamination during slaughter and fabrication complicate modeling and limit its ability to predict outcomes.

The committee recommends that the impact of data deficiencies and difficulties associated with data collection, which have been recognized in various parts of the FSIS draft risk assessment document, be more strongly emphasized in discussions of the outcomes calculated by the model. The data deficiencies identified by the risk assessment should serve as the foundation for a delineation of research priorities to be promoted or pursued so that the model (and *E. coli* O157:H7 policy decisions) can be improved in the future.

The committee also recommends that the authors add a discussion of the appropriate and inappropriate applications of the slaughter module in its present state of development—in particular, whether the module is ready to be used to draw conclusions about the factors most important in influencing the occurrence and extent of *E. coli* O157:H7 contamination in ground beef and the possible impact of interventions.

SOURCES OF CONTAMINATION AND CROSS CONTAMINATION DURING SLAUGHTER AND FABRICATION

Issues Regarding Fecal and Hide Contamination

The FSIS draft risk assessment states that "the number of *E. coli* O157:H7 organisms that initially contaminate a carcass depends on the level of infected cattle." However, carcass contamination (during dehiding and later steps) may originate not only from "infected" cattle but also from other sources, such as animal hides that cross-contaminate noninfected cattle during transportation, in holding areas, and during slaughter. In addition, carcasses and meat may become contaminated through O157:H7 niches that are established in plants and through cross contamination, not only during dehiding but also in handling at later stages of slaughter and fabrication (Samelis et al., 2002a).

As noted in the review of the Production Module, using fecal prevalence in slaughtered cattle as the *sole* measure of carcass contamination is a major weakness of the draft model. The FSIS draft risk assessment acknowledges that cross contamination may occur and notes that the hide is an additional source of contamination. The draft's justifications for using fecal contamination as the only source of carcass contamination are in the discussion of the knock box and stunning operations: there are sparse data on hide prevalence, the contribution of hide contamination is implicit in the existing model, and research indicates that the fecal status of incoming cattle correlates most strongly with carcass contamination.

Not considering potential sources of carcass and meat contamination other than animals carrying the pathogen in their gastrointestinal systems simplifies modeling but has major drawbacks. Omitted factors include contamination from animal hides and the influence of variations in plant design, size, capacity, and operational procedures on extent of contamination.

The committee recommends that the final risk assessment emphasize these weaknesses of the model and state that the outcomes of the model need to be recalculated after additional data become available or state that the model cannot provide informative predictions at this stage of its development because of lack of data in key segments of the process.

Issues Regarding the Use of Limited Data to Determine Carcass Contamination

The research of Elder and colleagues (2000) is cited as the primary support for the notion that fecal *E. coli* O157:H7 prevalence data best predict the quantitative correlation between preharvest and postharvest contamination. However, a close reading of the paper reveals a more complex picture. The Elder et al. data indicated that prevalence in all fecal *and hide* samples was significantly correlated with prevalence of positive carcasses ($p = 0.001$) and that there was "no significant difference between the proportion of lots positive on fecal and hide samples and those positive on carcass samples ($p = 0.2207$)." The authors note that their data suggest a lack of association between hide prevalence and carcass contamination and that there appears to be a correlation between fecal prevalence and initial carcass contamination. However, a possible reason for these findings is the lower prevalence of *E. coli* O157:H7 on hides than in feces in the study. Those data do not preclude situations in which hide prevalence is higher than fecal prevalence, in which case carcass contamination may correlate better with hide contamination. In addition, existence of a higher correlation between fecal and carcass prevalence does not preclude hide contamination—irrespective of how low it is—as the source of direct contamination or cross contamination of carcasses or meat.

The observations summarized in Table 2 of Elder et al. (2000), outlined below, illustrate the complexity of the situation.

- A group of cattle from a single source (a "lot") with high fecal contamination (76.5%) and hide contamination (11.1%) yielded carcasses with 0% postprocessing contamination.
- A lot with 0% fecal and hide contamination yielded carcasses with 75% contamination before evisceration and 0% after processing.
- Fecal and hide prevalence of 12.5% and 6.3% were associated with 56.3% and 0% prevalences in carcasses before evisceration and after processing, respectively.
- Fecal and hide prevalences of 11.1% and 77.8% were associated with 55.6% and 0% prevalences before and after evisceration, respectively.
- Fecal and hide prevalences of 0% and 50% were associated with 30% and 0% prevalences before and after evisceration, respectively.
- Some lots had 0% prevalence throughout the slaughtering process.
- Of the 29 lots sampled, 21 were positive for feces and 11 for hides; of the 30 at the carcass stage, 26 were positive before evisceration, 17 after evisceration, and 5 after processing.

Those observations confirm that contamination originates in feces and hides as well as from cross contamination (even if animal testing yields zero prevalence); hide removal is the most important operation that results in exposure of carcasses to contamination; slaughter-plant operations after dehiding, including decontamination processes, reduce contamination greatly, in terms of both lot and sample prevalence; and carcass contamination before evisceration, after evisceration, and especially after processing does not correlate well with fecal or hide contamination. Prevalence varies with animal lot and slaughter plant irrespective of extent of animal contamination, and decontamination greatly reduces pathogen prevalence.

The lack of higher correlation between hide and carcass prevalence in the Elder et al. study may alternatively or additionally be due to sampling limitations. The authors found the relatively low hide prevalence to be surprising and noted that "preliminary studies had indicated good concordance in isolation rates between fecal and hide samples on individual cattle." They state:

> One explanation for this apparent discrepancy is choice of sampling site [and it] is possible that other sites on the hide have higher levels of contamination, and are, therefore, greater risks for generating direct or airborne carcass contamination. It is also possible that survival rates of EHEC O157[1] differ by site on the hide. It is clear that hides do contribute to the total bacterial load, which may contribute to carcass contamination. Further studies are required to address the relative importance of hides as a source of carcass contamination by EHEC O157.

A more recent study by Ransom et al. (2002) supports that observation, finding that *E. coli* O157:H7 hide prevalence varied from 13.3% to 23.3%, depending on the method of sampling.

In summary, a limitation of the model—admittedly due to lack of data—is overreliance on a single study in the Slaughter Module—Elder et al. (2000). **The committee suggests that consideration be given to using available data on other pathogenic or indicator organisms to estimate proportional transfer of contamination (prevalence and levels) from live animals and the plant environment to carcasses during dehiding and possibly during later steps of the process. The committee also suggests that future studies be promoted to provide improved data for this part of the model.**

The Effect of Slaughter-Plant Methods on Cross Contamination of Carcasses

The FSIS draft risk assessment states that cross contamination of hides may occur in the knock box as noncontaminated cattle fall to the floor or come into contact with sides of the chute after contaminated cattle have passed through. It also cites literature that finds that additional contamination can occur if cattle emit feces or rumen contents at the knock box or if dirty knives are used. Thus, cross contamination is expected to occur, but it is difficult to predict. Data from studies by Elder et al. (2000), Bacon et al. (1999, 2000), and Ransom et al. (2002) indicate that the extent of contamination of live animals and carcasses immediately after hide removal and after carcass washing or chilling varies greatly among plants. That suggests that there is no obvious correlation between animal con-

---

[1] "EHEC [Enterohemorrhagic *Escherichia coli*] O157" is an alternative way to refer to the pathogen and is used in some scientific papers.

tamination and carcass contamination, especially after processing and in individual animal lots. Depending on the plant, lot, or time of slaughter, heavily contaminated cattle may be linked with high or low numbers of contaminated carcasses or with carcasses showing no detectable *E. coli* O157:H7 contamination. Slaughter-plant characteristics and operations clearly have an important influence on carcass contamination (irrespective of the extent of live-animal contamination), extent of cross contamination, and the effectiveness of decontamination. Thus, slaughter plants may influence contamination levels in ways that are not captured by the cow-bull versus steer-heifer modeling performed in the draft risk assessment.

Cross Contamination of the Carcass During Evisceration

The FSIS draft risk assessment identifies evisceration as a step in the slaughter process in which contamination may be introduced through unintentional perforation of the gastrointestinal tract. Although the draft asserts that "studies indicate that evisceration is usually carried out with minimal contamination," opportunities for additional contamination, cross-contamination, and spreading of contamination exist during evisceration and may vary with plant operations.

Although contamination and cross contamination originating in leakage of intestinal contents during evisceration are expected, available data on their extent are sparse or inadequate, and the cross-contaminating effect may be unpredictable. The draft cites a personal communication within the US Department of Agriculture (USDA) as the sole support for the assumption that gastrointestinal tract perforation potentially occurs in 1% of carcasses. Even if that rate of perforation, or leakage, is an underestimate, setting its probability between 0% and 2%, as the draft does, is almost certainly appropriate. **The committee notes that the cross contamination and redistribution of contamination that may occur at this stage (and other stages of the slaughter process) may at times be substantial and suggests that the final risk assessment explicitly acknowledge this.**

Factoring in Cross Contamination During Processing

The Elder et al. (2000) paper clearly indicates that cross contamination occurs during processing. It notes that "the overall prevalence of carcass contamination with EHEC O157 was significantly greater than that of fecal and hide prevalence" and that carcass samples in the same lot were positive even when no animals were fecal- or hide-positive. And the FSIS draft risk assessment recognizes the importance of self-contamination and cross contamination in several places, acknowledging that "the exterior surface of the hide and the environment in the dehiding area are recognized sources of pathogens (Grau, 1987)" and that "cross-contamination can occur via workers' gloves, knives, clothing, or during the changing of the hide-puller from one carcass to the next (Gill et al., 1999)."[2]

It can be argued that by estimating the frequency of contaminated carcasses at 120% and 160% of the prevalence of incoming contaminated cattle during the low- and high-prevalence seasons, respectively, the draft model is in effect factoring in cross contamination. However, the distributions around the values need to be based on more data. The calculation of the low-prevalence season figure is particularly problematic. It is derived by creating a "mixture" of the high-prevalence season transformation ratio and a uniform distribution ranging from near 0 to a maximum of the high-season ratio. **The committee suggests that the risk assessment emphasize the need for additional data so that the frequency of cross contamination can be estimated with more confidence in later refinements of the model.**

Issues Regarding Cross Contamination During Fabrication

There is a need for data to attempt to estimate the frequency and extent of cross contamination during fabrication, although this would be a difficult, costly, and time-consuming undertaking and could yield results of great uncertainty. As stated by Newton et al. (1978), "structural and work surfaces may be as important as the hide as sources of bacterial contamination of meat." To deal with the lack of data, the FSIS draft model relies on output data from the grinder segment of the Preparation Module, and it appears that inputs were adjusted to fit expectations. **The committee suggests that consideration be given to whether it could be more appropriate to adjust inputs at previous stages of the model (for example, with data on prevalence in carcasses in the chiller) to predict contamination better.**

Issues Regarding the Accuracy with Which Data Were Copied from Sources

A transformation ratio (TR) is used in the FSIS draft risk assessment to relate the frequency of contaminated carcasses to the frequency of cattle in a lot carrying the pathogen. The fraction of carcasses contaminated

---

[2] A later paper by Gill et al. (2001), published after the draft risk assessment was released, documents cross contamination from equipment during carcass splitting in greater detail.

during dehiding is based on the results of the study of Elder et al. (2000) that reports on cattle and carcass prevalences in four slaughter plants during July–August 1999. Concerns associated with the calculation of those variables include the use of a single study for such an important part of the model (it is recognized that there is little research on the topic) and the observation that there are discrepancies in the numbers cited in the draft risk assessment and Elder et al. (2000). Specifically, the draft risk assessment states: "In lots showing evidence of *E. coli* O157:H7 in cattle or on carcasses, 91 of 307 [327 according to Elder et al. (2000)] cattle (30% [28%]) and 148 of 312 [341 according to Elder et al.] carcasses at dehiding (47% [43%]) were *E. coli* O157:H7 positive." The independent review by Edmund Crouch in Appendix D notes additional concerns with the calculation of the TR for the low prevalence season.

The committee recommends that the numbers found in the FSIS draft risk assessment and attendant model be cross-checked for accuracy with the data presented in the published study of Elder et al. (2000).

LEVELS AND EXTENT OF SURFACE-AREA CONTAMINATION

The FSIS draft risk assessment, citing Galland (1997), notes that the number of *E. coli* O157:H7 organisms that initially contaminate a carcass and the level of infected cattle are affected by the average concentration of organisms per unit contaminated area and the total area of a carcass that is contaminated. However, it acknowledges that no published information is available on those factors. Collecting data to develop estimates (especially for the total surface area of the carcass and trim that is contaminated) may be difficult, but an informative model needs to account for the factors that greatly affect the extent of contamination.

Issues Regarding Contamination of the Carcass During Dehiding (Step 2)

To estimate the number of *E. coli* O157:H7 organisms on a contaminated carcass, it is necessary to know the number of organisms per square centimeter and the total contaminated surface area of the carcass. As the draft risk assessment notes, however, there is a lack of data on both those variables. The lack of information was handled in the draft by using data from a study conducted by the USDA Food Safety and Inspection Service (FSIS) in 1994. In that study, carcass surface tissue was excised after carcass chilling in plants throughout the United States and shipped to laboratories for analysis of various microorganisms, including *E. coli* O157:H7. Samples of 60 cm^2 were taken from carcasses originating in feedlots. Of 2,081 samples tested, four were positive for *E. coli* O157:H7: two at less than 0.03 CFU/cm² and two at 0.301–3.0 CFU/cm². That information was used to estimate the number of *E. coli* O157:H7 organisms on a contaminated carcass at dehiding. The data were combined with sampling information from the Elder et al. (2000) study—in which 6 of 330 carcass samples taken at the post-processing stage tested positive for O157:H7—to form a ratio that was used to adjust the FSIS figures for contamination below the detection limit of that study.

The committee notes several weaknesses associated with that approach: the number of samples found positive was extremely small; the positive samples were analyzed after carcass chilling, at which point the contamination density may have been reduced by carcass washing and chilling, compared with the density at dehiding; the surface area analyzed was sampled with two methods—tissue excision in the 1994 FSIS study and swabbing in the Elder et al. (2000) study; the studies used different analytic methods; and, the amount of carcass surface area sampled and analyzed was much smaller in the FSIS study (60 cm²) than in the Elder et al. study (450 cm²). It also observes that available information on the confidence interval around the percentage of positive samples in the Elder et al. study (listed in Table 1 of the paper) was not used.

On the basis of those observations, the committee believes that the weaknesses render the calculation of the adjustment ratio problematic and raise questions about the reliability of the estimates derived from the analysis. **The committee recommends that these weaknesses be highlighted and the need for additional data be emphasized in the risk assessment.**

Issues Regarding the Difficulties of Determining Surface Contamination

Lack of information on the surface area contaminated is also of concern. The FSIS draft authors manage it by subjectively setting the minimum area of contamination at 30 cm² and the maximum area at 3,000 cm² because "initial model runs showed that contaminated surface areas greater than 3,000 cm² produced results that were infeasible in comparison with FSIS ground beef sampling data." The range of contamination density predicted with those assumptions is 1 to 9,000 cells.

The committee acknowledges that such data are difficult to obtain or predict and that contamination of the carcass surface is expected to be localized, nonuniform, random, and nonhomogeneous, and notes that the range of contamination density predicted may well be wide enough to account for all the unknowns in the calculation. However, it points out that the derivation of the values in the draft is arbitrary and unscientific. **The committee suggests that one potential approach to deal with** concerns about determining surface contamination may be to use available data on density and extent of carcass contamination with indicator organisms, such as *E. coli* biotype I. The draft risk assessment notes that Bell (1997), reporting on New Zealand operations, measured densities of generic *E. coli* on carcasses. In addition to those results, data from several studies of North American plants may be useful in the estimation (for example, Bacon et al., 2000; Gill et al., 1996a,b; Graves Delmore et al., 1997, 1998; Reagan et al., 1996; Sofos et al., 1999a,b,c,d; Van Donkersgoed et al. 1997). Some of those studies and others report data at several steps in the slaughtering process that might be useful in estimating proportional transfer and cell density on carcasses. **Future studies could be proposed to provide better data for the improvement of this part of the model.**

Issues Regarding the Effects of the First (Step 3) and Second (Step 5) Decontamination on Prevalence, Levels, and Extent of Contamination

Decontamination is modeled at two points in the draft Slaughter Module: a first decontamination after dehiding (Step 3) and a second after carcass splitting (Step 5). The committee has several observations and suggestions concerning those steps.

First Decontamination

The committee notes that not all plants apply a first decontamination; this should be explicitly recognized in the risk assessment. The FSIS draft notes that a variety of organic acids are used for decontamination, but it does not specify which, if any, are in common use. The committee observes that lactic and, to a lesser extent, acetic acid are used. It also observes that the use of hot water cited in the draft may be limited before evisceration because of potential condensate formation.

Gill (1999) and Dorsa et al. (1997) are cited to justify the range of most-likely log reductions due to first decontamination—0.3 and 0.7, respectively. However, the draft fails to justify the choice of the range of maximal values used—0.8–1.2; they might simply be 0.5 log additions to the "most-likely" values. **The committee recommends that the risk assessment delineate how the maximal magnitudes of contamination reduction were determined.**

The draft states that "while visible signs of foreign matter can be readily identified and removed, bacterial colonies themselves are not directly observable." It should be pointed out that bacteria on carcasses shortly after dehiding are probably not in the form of colonies, but instead in the form of cells or clusters of cells that are not macroscopically visible. The term *colony* typically refers to a mass of cells that is formed by multiplication of single cells or clumps of cells on a nutrient agar plate or a stored product and that is macroscopically visible.

The draft report needs to clarify whether the "total outside surface area" of a carcass includes the area of the body cavity, which is also exposed to the environment and may be contaminated during evisceration or after carcass splitting.

The committee notes two factors that are not reflected in the draft's first-decontamination model:

- The extent of decontamination may also be affected by level (density) of initial contamination, especially when "hot" (highly contaminated) spots exist on a carcass (Graves Delmore et al., 1998; Dorsa, 1997; Smulders and Greer, 1998; Sofos and Smith, 1998).
- Initial contamination by knives, gloves, and other equipment is noted in the text as a potential source. However, the draft does not allow for the possibility of an increase in contamination at this step.

The committee recommends that these omissions be at least acknowledged as weaknesses in the model.

Second Decontamination

The committee believes that several details regarding the second decontamination ought to be better reflected in the text:

- The second decontamination step is applied after "zero tolerance" carcass inspection[3] and any associated trimming or steam vacuuming that may be necessary to meet "zero tolerance" inspection requirements.
- The procedures used for the second decontamination depend not only on the size of the plant, as stated in the draft risk assessment, but also on such factors as equipment availability, costs, plant design, space available, and steam availability.
- All plants use knife trimming and some type of water rinsing or spraying, but steam pasteurization is not used universally (although it is quite common).

---

[3] The requirements for zero tolerance carcass inspection are addressed in FSIS Directive 6420.1: Livestock Post-Mortem Inspection Activities–Enforcing the Zero Tolerances for Fecal Material, Ingesta, and Ilk (December 17, 1998). In brief, it requires the removal of feces, ingesta, and udder contents from beef carcasses, by trimming, before carcass washing as a means of improving the cleanliness and microbiological status of beef.

- The use of steam pasteurization, hot-water rinsing (thermal pasteurization), and organic-acid rinsing varies among plants, depending on the factors mentioned above.
- A number of references in addition to Bell (1997) have reported on the results of decontamination interventions. These include Bacon et al. (2000); Bolton et al. (2001); Graves Delmore et al. (1997, 1998); Nutsch et al. (1997, 1998); Reagan et al. (1996). Such references should be consulted to determine whether they could better inform the modeling of this step.
- The efficacy of decontamination procedures depends on such factors as pressure, temperature, cabinet or chamber design, nozzle configuration and operation, and length of application.
- The assumption that "large plants typically use a steam pasteurization process" is not entirely correct, in that some large plants use hot-water or organic-acid rinses after carcass washing.
- The draft states that "Phebus et al. (1997) found 3.53 ± 0.49 log CFU/cm^2 reduction in $E.\ coli$ O157:H7 on inoculated carcasses." It should be clarified that those authors evaluated carcass samples inoculated with over 5 logs and that the reduction was achieved after 15 seconds of steam pasteurization, which is about twice as long as practical applications. It should be noted that findings with inocula in experimental circumstances can be very different from those with natural flora in commercial circumstances.
- Two Nutsch et al. papers (1997, 1998) are cited to support the statement that "other studies have shown reductions in prevalence of $E.\ coli$ O157:H7-contaminated carcasses from steam pasteurization." The cited studies evaluated carcasses in plants but not $E.\ coli$ O157:H7; they involved nonpathogenic contaminants.

The committee suggests that these observations be considered in revising the FSIS risk assessment to provide a more complete depiction of plant operations. However, it notes that the wide variations in practices for second decontamination may not necessarily result in substantially different reductions in contamination.

The FSIS draft states that "given standard industry behavior and available evidence, variability in steam pasteurization efficacy... was modeled using triangular distribution with a minimum value of 0 logs, an uncertain most-likely value of 0.5 to 1.5 logs, and an uncertain maximum value of 1.51 to 2.5 logs." Those values appear reasonable, but **the committee recommends that the risk assessment explicitly state the reasoning underlying them and note, if appropriate, that they apply not only to steam pasteurization but also to other methods applied individually or in combination in carcass decontamination.**

The FSIS draft factors in the effect of decontamination on cell density (specifically, the log reduction in cell density). **The committee suggests that consideration be given to the effects of decontamination on pathogen prevalence and the contaminated surface area.** In general, although data available on potential changes in contamination loads (cell densities) and contaminated surface area are sparse or nonexistent, data on the prevalence of *E. coli* O157:H7 on carcasses after decontamination and chilling are available (Elder et al., 2000 and others). **The committee suggests that the importance of these variables in model development be acknowledged, reconsidered, and explained.**

TERMINOLOGY CONCERNS

As noted elsewhere in this review, the FSIS draft risk assessment sometimes defines or uses terms in nonstandard ways. The committee found a few circumstances in the Slaughter Module in which that might confuse readers.

The draft risk assessment defines *trim* as a *byproduct* of processing carcasses to create cuts of meat (such as steaks and roasts) when the carcasses originate as feedlot cattle and as the *primary product* that results from deboning carcasses that originate as breeding cattle. Trim is not necessarily a byproduct, considering its volume and value. The meat industry considers such items as intestines, tongues, livers, and stomachs to be byproducts. Although a major proportion of cows and bulls becomes trim, a substantial amount is also used for less expensive steaks or in roast-beef production.

Later, in the discussion of fabrication, the expression *leftover trim* is used. It is confusing because trim is by definition what is left after primal cuts are removed. The text should also make it clear that only a small amount of such trim is typically vacuum packaged.

Lot is defined in the draft as the number of cattle necessary to fill one combo bin with trim; and a single lot may take one or more truckloads of cattle. To avoid potential confusion, it should be explained that in slaughter operations a lot is typically defined as a group of animals for slaughter that have a common source (a ranch or feedlot, for example) and are slaughtered together. The latter definition is used, for example, in the Elder et al. (2000) paper. During fabrication, the industry may consider product that moves from one cleanup operation to the next as a lot.

Plants are modeled as those which slaughter culled cows and bulls, called "breeding cattle", and those which slaughter cattle fed in feedlots, called "feedlot cattle". These terms, used throughout the exposure assessment, might not be the most appropriate choices, because they are somewhat misleading. For example, dairy animals, which are in the "breeding" category, are not breeding. Potential alternative terms are *fed* or *feeder* steers or heifers versus *non-fed, cull, mature,* or *market* cows or bulls.

In the discussion of the transportation segment, the term *susceptible cattle* is used. It is not defined, and it is not clear what the authors are referring to.

The committee suggests that the authors either adopt new terminology that clearly states concepts and definitions or align their definitions with those conventionally used in risk assessments to minimize confusion and misunderstanding. The review of the draft's risk characterization (in Chapter 6) also addresses this point.

OTHER OBSERVATIONS

The FSIS draft risk assessment models cows and bulls separately from steers and heifers because most operations slaughter one of the two groups of animals. However, as indicated in the draft, a small number of plants (perhaps two to four) slaughter both types of animals. If those plants are excluded from the model, that should be explicitly acknowledged and the decision explicated.

The draft states (p. 59) that the probability and extent of *E. coli* O157:H7 contamination or decontamination during slaughter are modeled as dependent on

- the status of the incoming animal (separate variables for the numbers of infected breeding and feedlot cattle arriving at slaughter in a truck and extent of contamination),
- the type of slaughter plant (modeled indirectly—breeding and feedlot cattle are presumed to be sent to separate plants),
- the type of equipment and procedures used (implicitly modeled—different types of decontamination are assumed for large versus small plants—hot water versus steam—and different efficacies are associated with them,
- the efficacy of decontamination procedures (separately modeled for large versus small plants), and
- the sanitation processes (which may be implicitly modeled via the efficacy of decontamination techniques, although this is not explicitly stated).

The text does not mention whether those variables are included as factors in the model or simply considered to be included through the assumptions made in developing the model. It is true that there are few data available for determining the roles of most of, if not all, these variables. **However, such factors as plant design and capacity, specific combina-**

tions of decontamination interventions used, and efficacy of sanitation procedures may be highly influential in carcass contamination, and the committee recommends that the text make their role in the model more clear.

More generally, the draft considers seven steps of the slaughter process. It indicates that the slaughter process contains other steps but that they are not explicitly modeled. Although the role of the steps omitted may not be easy to predict or model, depending on the plant, the steps may be important in cross contamination, so their roles should be better acknowledged in the text.

In the "Arrival" step (1), the proportions of weight that amounts to trim from cow carcasses (53%) and bull carcasses (90%) may have been overestimated, considering that sizable amounts of these carcasses may be used for lower-priced steak and roast-beef items. Furthermore, although the FSIS draft risk assessment states that those values represent midpoints of uncertainty distributions that "can range ±20%" (p. 61), the draft's Appendix C states that the variable representing the proportion (ρ) is deterministic rather than stochastic (p. 174). The risk assessment must clarify whether the variability identified in the text is actually reflected in the model.

The Arrival step discussion also indicates that the number of combo bins to which a steer or heifer carcass contributes trim depends on the number of trim "sortings," which is based on fat content. That needs to be acknowledged in the risk assessment; if it is not modeled, a reason should be provided.

The discussion of carcass fabrication (Step 7) indicates that "Scanga et al. (2000) found no difference in the concentration of *E. coli* O157:H7 across fat content" in different types of beef trimmings. It should be clarified that those authors did not analyze for *E. coli* O157:H7 (which was considered an adulterant). However, they found higher bacterial counts and prevalence of other pathogens in trimmings as the fat content increased.

Although the draft discussion of contamination from a single carcass states that the amount of O157:H7 contamination in a combo bin depends on the number of contaminated carcasses and the amount of contamination that each carcass contributes, a major factor in the contamination of individual combo bins may be redistribution of contamination and cross contamination during fabrication. That unmodeled factor may in turn be affected by plant size, plant procedures and design, animal type, and the like.

The committee is aware of research on the impact of seasonal variation and other factors on the incidence of *E. coli* O157 and *Salmonella* in slaughter facilities being sponsored by the National Cattlemen's Beef Association. These results, when available, may help to fill some of the data gaps identified here.

SUMMARY REMARKS

In summary, the FSIS draft risk assessment correctly acknowledges that published data on E. coli O157:H7 prevalence and levels (cell density) during slaughter and fabrication are scarce. In addition, data on the surface area contaminated and the extent of cross contamination are lacking. One reason for the paucity of published data may be the status of E. coli O157:H7 as an adulterant in ground beef and other nonintact beef products; this may have discouraged studies of the detection of E. coli O157:H7 in fresh beef. The draft recognizes the importance of data by stating that the occurrence and extent of carcass contamination, effectiveness of decontamination procedures, and effect of carcass chilling are among the factors that most influence the occurrence and extent of E. coli O157:H7 contamination in ground beef. It also recognizes the scarcity of available data and the need for more research to obtain additional information on the contribution of the hide to carcass contamination; on the prevalence, extent, and density of E. coli O157:H7 contamination on carcasses after dehiding; on the contribution of cross contamination to product contamination; on the effect of carcass decontamination and chilling on increases or decreases in E. coli O157:H7 organisms; and on the influence of fabrication activities on redistribution of contamination in meat cuts and trimmings. The correlation analysis presented as part of the sensitivity analysis indicates that the E. coli O157:H7-contaminated carcass surface area and the effects of carcass chilling have the greatest influence on the occurrence of the pathogen in combo bins and grinder loads. However, the lack of publicly available data on crucial steps in the slaughter process, the variability of the operations modeled in the Slaughter Module, and the potential unpredictability of the effects of some activities on contamination during slaughter and carcass fabrication complicate modeling and limit the module's predictive capacity.

The lack of data has made development of the model difficult and has created the necessity to rely heavily on the results of one study (Elder et al., 2000) to make major assumptions, and to adjust some inputs to fit the expected outcomes of the model. Although assumptions are often necessary in model development, the committee recommends that those difficulties and deficiencies be more strongly emphasized in discussions of the outcomes calculated by the model and that the need for more data for model improvement be highlighted throughout the report, including in the Conclusions, the Executive Summary, and the Interpretive Summary. Furthermore, the committee recommends that the report stress the potential influence of some plant activities on cross contamination, on the level of contamination, and on the extent of carcass or trim surface area contaminated. It must be made clear that the impact of those activities, although important, may be difficult to characterize empirically. The committee thus recommends that the authors add a discussion of the appropriate and inappropriate applications of the model in its present state of development—in particular, whether the Slaughter Module is ready to be used to draw conclusions about the factors most important in the occurrence and extent of *E. coli* O157:H7 contamination in ground beef and the possible impact of interventions. The committee thus suggests that the report explicitly recognize that the myriad factors that influence *E. coli* O157:H7 presence, spread, growth, and elimination throughout the slaughter process are at present very difficult to characterize empirically. This means that model limitations must be acknowledged, that alternative approaches such as using data on other pathogenic or indicator organisms be considered for use in the short term, and that research priorities identified in the risk assessment be promoted or pursued so that the model can be improved in the future.

REFERENCES

Bacon RT, Belk KE, Sofos JN, Smith GC. 1999. Incidence of *Escherichia coli* O157:H7 on hide, carcass and beef trimmings samples collected from United States packing plants. Proceedings of the 53rd Annual Reciprocal Meat Conference. pp. 106–108.

Bacon RT, Belk KE, Sofos JN, Clayton RP, Reagan JO, Smith GC. 2000. Microbial populations on animal hides and beef carcasses at different stages of slaughter in plants employing multiple-sequential interventions for decontamination. Journal of Food Protection 63:1080–1086.

Bell RG. 1997. Distribution and sources of microbial contamination on beef carcasses. Journal of Applied Microbiology 82:292–300.

Bolton DJ, Doherty AM, Sheridan JJ. 2001. Beef HACCP: Intervention and non-intervention systems. International Journal of Food Microbiology 66(1-2):119–129.

Dorsa WJ. 1997. New and established carcass decontamination procedures commonly used in the beef-processing industry. Journal of Food Protection 60(9):1146–1151.

Dorsa WJ, Cutter CN, Siragusa GR. 1997. Effects of acetic acid, lactic acid and trisodium phosphate on the microflora of refrigerated beef carcass surface tissue inoculated with *Escherichia coli* O157:H7, *Listeria innocua*, and *Clostridium sporogenes*. Journal of Food Protection 60(6):619–624.

Elder RO, Keen JE, Siragusa GR, Barkocy-Gallagher GA, Koohmaraie M, Laegreid WW. 2000. Correlation of enterohemorrhagic *Escherichia coli* O157 prevalence in feces, hides, and carcasses of beef cattle during processing. Proceedings of the National Academy of Sciences 97(7):2999–3003.

FSIS (Food Safety and Inspection Service). 1994. Nationwide Beef Microbiological Baseline Data Collection Program: Steers and Heifers—October 1992–September 1993.

Galland JC. 1997. Risks and prevention of contamination of beef carcasses during the slaughter process in the United States of America. Revue scientifique et technique (International Office of Epizootics) 16(2):395–404.

Gill CO. 1999. HACCP by guesswork or by the numbers? Food Quality (January/February). pp. 28–32.

Gill CO, Badoni M, Jones T. 1996a. Hygienic effects of trimming and washing operations in a beef-carcass-dressing process. Journal of Food Protection 59(6):666–669.

Gill CO, McGinniss J, Badoni M. 1996b. Assessment of the hygienic characteristics of a beef carcass dressing process. Journal of Food Protection 59(2):136–140.

Gill CO, Badoni M, McGinnis JC. 1999. Assessment of the adequacy of cleaning of equipment used for breaking beef carcasses. International Journal of Food Microbiology 46(1):1–8.

Gill CO, McGinnis JC, Bryant J. 2001. Contamination of beef chucks with *Escherichia coli* during carcass breaking. Journal of Food Protection 64(11):1824–1827.

Grau FH. 1987. Prevention of microbial contamination in the export beef abattoir. In: Smulders FJM, ed. Elimination of Pathogenic Organisms from Meat and Poultry. Amsterdam: Elsevier Press, pp. 221–223.

Graves Delmore LR, Sofos JN, Reagan JO, Smith GC. 1997. Hot-water rinsing and trimming/washing of beef carcasses to reduce physical and microbiological contamination. Journal of Food Science 62:373–376.

Graves Delmore LR, Sofos JN, Schmidt GR, Smith GC. 1998. Decontamination of inoculated beef with sequential spraying treatments. Journal of Food Science 63:890–893.

Newton KG, Harrison JCL, Wauters AM. 1978. Sources of psychrotrophic bacteria on meat at the abattoir. Journal of Applied Bacteriology 45:75–82.

Nutsch AL, Phebus RK, Riemann MJ, Schafer DE, Boyer JE Jr, Wilson RC, Leising JD, Kastner CL. 1997. Evaluation of a steam pasteurization process in a commercial beef processing facility. Journal of Food Protection 60:485–492.

Nutsch AL, Phebus RK, Riemann MJ, Kotrola JS, Wilson RC, Boyer JE Jr, Brown TL. 1998. Steam pasteurization of commercially slaughtered beef carcasses: evaluation of bacterial populations at five anatomical locations. Journal of Food Protection 61:571–577.

Phebus RD, Nutsch AL, Schafer DE, Wilson RC, Riemann MJ, Leising JD, Kastner CL, Wolf JR, Prasai RK. 1997. Comparison of steam pasteurization and other methods for reduction of pathogens on surfaces of freshly slaughtered beef. Journal of Food Protection 60:476–484.

Ransom JR, Belk KE, Bacon RT, Sofos JN, Scanga JA, Smith GC. 2002. Comparison of sampling methods for microbiological testing of beef animal rectal/colonal feces, hides and carcasses. Journal of Food Protection 65(4):621–626.

Reagan JO, Acuff GR, Buege DR, Buyck MJ, Dickson JS, Kastner CL, Marsden JL, Morgan JB, Nickelson R II, Smith GC, Sofos JN. 1996. Trimming and washing of beef carcasses as a method of improving the microbiological quality of meat. Journal of Food Protection 59:751–756.

Samelis J, Sofos JN, Kendal PA, Smith GC. 2001a. Influence of the natural microbial flora on acid tolerance response of *Listeria monocytogenes* in a model system of fresh meat decontamination fluids. Applied and Environmental Microbiology 67:2410–2420.

Samelis J, Sofos JN, Kendall PA, Smith GC. 2001b. Fate of *Escherichia coli* O157:H7, *Salmonella* Typhimurium DT104 and *Listeria monocytogenes* in fresh meat decontamination fluids at 4 and 10°C. Journal of Food Protection 64:950–957.

Samelis J, Sofos JN, Kendall PA, Smith GC. 2002a. Effect of acid adaptation on survival of *Escherichia coli* O157:H7 in meat decontamination washing fluids, and potential effects of organic acid interventions on the microbial ecology of the meat plant environment. Journal of Food Protection 65(1):33–40.

Samelis J, Sofos JN, Ikeda JS, Kendall PA, Smith GC. 2002b. Exposure to water meat decontamination washing fluids sensitizes *Escherichia coli* O157:H7 to organic acids. Letters in Applied Microbiology 34:7–12.

Scanga JA, Grona AD, Belk KE, Sofos JN, Bellinger GR, Smith GC. 2000. Microbiological contamination of raw beef trimmings and ground beef. Meat Science 56:145–152.

Smulders FJM, Greer GG. 1998. Integrating microbial decontamination with organic acids in HACCP programmes for muscle foods: Prospects and controversies. International Journal of Food Microbiology 44:149–169.

Sofos JN, Smith GC. 1998. Nonacid meat decontamination technologies: Model studies and commercial applications. International Journal of Food Microbiology 44:171–188.

Sofos JN, Belk KE, Smith GC. 1999a. Processes to reduce contamination with pathogenic microorganisms in meat. Proceedings of the 45th International Congress of Meat Science and Technology (Japan). Vol. II, pp. 596–605.

Sofos JN, Kochevar SL, Bellinger GR, Buege DR, Hancock DD, Ingham SC, Morgan JB, Reagan JO, Smith GC. 1999b. Sources and extent of microbiological contamination of beef carcasses in seven United States slaughtering plants. Journal of Food Protection 62:140–145.

Sofos JN, Kochevar SL, Reagan JO, Smith GC. 1999c. Extent of beef carcass contamination with *Escherichia coli* and probabilities of passing U.S. regulatory criteria. Journal of Food Protection 62:234–238.

Sofos JN, Kochevar SL, Reagan JO, Smith GC. 1999d. Incidence of *Salmonella* on beef carcasses relating to the U.S. meat and poultry inspection regulations. Journal of Food Protection 62:467–473.

Van Donkersgoed J, Jericho KWF, Grogan H, Thorlakson B. 1997. Preslaughter hide status of cattle and the microbiology of carcasses. Journal of Food Protection 60:1502–1508.

4

Preparation Module

The purpose of the Preparation Module is to estimate the occurrence and extent of *E. coli* O157:H7 contamination in consumed ground-beef servings. The approach involves determining the frequency of exposure of consumers in different age groups to *E. coli* O157:H7 in ground beef served at and away from home. Six primary steps are evaluated: grinding of beef, ground-beef storage during processing or by the retailer or distributor; transportation to the home or to hotels, restaurants, and institutions (HRI); storage at home or in HRI; cooking; and consumption. Consumption patterns are modeled as being dependent on the age of the consumer and the location of the meal. Ground beef is consumed in many forms, but the FSIS draft risk assessment focuses on hamburger patties and on ground beef used as a major ingredient in beef-based foods (such as meatballs and meatloaf). The model does not include ground beef as a granulated ingredient (as in commercial meat sauce for spaghetti).

CROSS CONTAMINATION

A central issue for the committee in its review of the draft Preparation Module was the factoring in of the contributing influence of cross contamination on human illness. Cross contamination during preparation results when *E. coli* O157:H7 is transmitted from contaminated ground beef to such vehicles as other foods, food preparation and processing surfaces, and food handlers. Because of the highly infectious nature of the pathogen, which has an estimated low infectious dose of under 100 cells, vehicles cross-contaminated through direct or indirect exposure to *E. coli*

O157:H7-tainted raw ground beef are likely to be important sources of human illness (Buchanan and Doyle, 1997).

A case-control analysis of sporadic infection with *E. coli* O157:H7 by Mead et al. (1997) substantiates that notion. It determined that most ill persons in question had eaten hamburgers prepared at home and that the primary risk factors associated with infection were food preparers who had not washed their hands or work surfaces after handling raw ground beef. The investigators concluded that in many instances hamburgers were not the direct vehicle of transmission of *E. coli* O157:H7, but rather that transmission occurred more commonly when the food preparers' hands, contaminated by raw ground beef, were allowed to cross-contaminate other meal items or utensils. In a multistate outbreak of *E. coli* O157:H7 infection in 1995, cross contamination from raw ground beef was identified as the likely contributing factor associated with eating cooked ground-beef sandwiches prepared at fast-food restaurants of a specific chain (CDC, 1996).

Although they did not address the issue of *E. coli* O157:H7 directly, two studies released while the draft risk assessment was under development support the notion that cross contamination during food preparation is an important risk factor for foodborne illness in general. Audits International (2001) published a study of food-preparation practices that identified cross contamination (25% of failures) as the third most-common critical violation[1] of good hygienic practices in the home. Previous Audits International studies had ranked it as the most common critical violation, with a frequency of 71% in 1997 and 31% in 1999. Another study researching commercial and institutional food operations was prepared by the Food and Drug Administration (FDA, 2000). Researchers at FDA found that 15% of fast-food restaurants and 44% of full-service restaurants examined were out of compliance with one or more items in the category "contaminated equipment/protection from contamination". Those items included whether raw animal foods were separated from one another, whether raw and ready-to-eat foods were separated, and whether surfaces and utensils were cleaned or sanitized.

The Food Safety and Inspection Service (FSIS) of the US Department of Agriculture (USDA) itself identifies cross contamination during preparation as a significant factor in food safety. Two of the four steps in USDA's Fight BAC!² campaign—"*Clean*—wash hands and surfaces often" and "*Separate*—don't cross-contaminate"—address interventions intended to minimize it.

---

[1] Critical violations are defined as conditions or actions that by themselves can cause foodborne illness.
[2] Where "BAC" refers to bacteria.

However, the FSIS draft risk assessment indicates that cross contamination in the preparation stage is outside the scope of the analysis (p. 3). Later (p.74), it states:

> Currently, quantitative modeling of cross-contamination in foods is hampered by a dearth of evidence. Furthermore, cross-contamination pathways are potentially complex, and each pathway may require as much data regarding growth dynamics and cooking effect as the primary product of interest. The model, however, can serve as a starting point for analyzing the effects of cross-contamination on human exposure to *E. coli* O157:H7.

The committee understands and respects the decision of the modelers to establish reasonable bounds on the reach of their work; it is a necessary part of any risk assessment. It observes, however, that cross contamination during preparation is an established, important risk factor; that the lack of data on its effects is no more severe than the lack of data for some other parts of the draft model; and that further attention to cross contamination will help to lay the groundwork for an analysis and better identify the data gaps that need to be filled by future research efforts.

The value of the risk assessment in informing public health policy and supporting regulatory interventions will be increased if it is able to factor in the effect of cross contamination on *E. coli* O157:H7 infections and perhaps address the influence of interventions. Just as important, the committee is concerned that the draft risk assessment may foster the inaccurate and misleading impression that proper cooking of ground beef will prevent all associated *E. coli* O157:H7 infections. If the model is used to simulate the effects of various interventions on human health outcomes, omission of this major route of infection could produce ambiguous results and potentially deficient policy decisions.

The committee recognizes that data are lacking on the extent to which various forms of exposure—whether direct (through contact with contaminated beef itself) or indirect (through contact with meat drippings or with surfaces that have previously been in contact with contaminated drippings or beef)—to *E. coli* O157:H7-tainted raw ground beef during storage, transportation, and meal-making affect infection. However, that is not the only circumstance in the FSIS draft model in which there is a dearth of information. As noted elsewhere in the chapter, for example, some estimates of the amount of raw ground beef consumed in subpopulations are derived from rather scanty data, and simplifying assumptions or conjectures are used in lieu of data in several steps of the Slaughter Module.

The committee also acknowledges that it may not now be possible to model cross contamination at a level of detail that would permit informed analysis of the efficacy of specific interventions. However, it points out that the ability to specify the particulars of the myriad scenarios by which cross contamination with raw ground beef can occur is not a prerequisite for accounting for this risk factor in the model. As noted elsewhere in this review, the process of constructing a risk assessment necessarily results in the identification of critical data gaps. With a better understanding of what information would be needed to perform more-sophisticated modeling, USDA will be in a better position to define a research agenda.

In summary, disregarding the contribution of cross contamination of *E. coli* O157:H7-tainted raw ground beef to human illness weakens the draft risk assessment. **The committee suggests that consideration be given to factoring in cross contamination as an additional step. If that is not possible, it recommends that the final FSIS risk assessment highlight more clearly the role of cross contamination in *E. coli* O157:H7 infection and emphasize the limitations in the model engendered by a decision to not factor it in.**

MODELING IN THE PREPARATION MODULE

Data Selected for Use and Means of Analysis Have Weaknesses

An important limitation in modeling in the Preparation Module is the paucity of adequate or validated data regarding some components of the preparation steps. It leads to diminished confidence in estimates derived from these data.

One example is the modeling of storage times. There are no data that directly document the length of time that ground beef is stored at refrigeration temperature. The draft uses storage temperature data of Audits International (1999) (Table 3-16 in the draft risk assessment) for home and HRI storage (Step 4). However, those data were obtained from a supermarket study in which temperatures were monitored from the retail distribution channel into the home, and it is inappropriate to extrapolate them to the whole of the HRI industry, because the vast majority of ground beef distributed through the food-service segment of HRI is distributed frozen. Such ground beef is processed into patties that are transported frozen and cooked from the frozen state. Hence, it is important to recognize that the Audits International data are relevant only to retail products and a minor portion of HRI ground beef. The vast majority of ground beef used in HRI is stored frozen, so the storage-temperature profiles of the product would be much different from those of fresh ground beef stored in a home setting.

The FSIS draft risk assessment does attempt to model the effects of freezing ground beef on *E. coli* O157:H7 cell numbers during storage and distribution (p. 83), assuming a uniform distribution of 20–80% of ground beef is produced frozen. That estimate, though, is so broad as to be uninformative. The committee suggests that expert opinion be sought regarding a more precise estimate and distribution and, if it is found useful, that it be documented in the text and used in the model until data become available. Any revised estimate should recognize that most ground-beef products used by the food-service sector are stored frozen.

The committee recommends, in general, that more precise information regarding the percentage of ground beef that is stored and distributed frozen and cooked from the frozen state be obtained and used for determining estimates associated with frozen ground beef, especially that used by fast-food restaurants. A trade association, such as the American Meat Institute, could be a source of this information.

Differences in Cooking Practices Based on Location Are Not Appropriately Considered

Practices for cooking ground beef in the home, at fast-food restaurants, and in other HRI facilities vary considerably; those of major chain fast-food restaurants are well defined and validated to kill pathogens, whereas those used in the home are based largely on the appearance of the cooked product and may result in pathogen survival. A 2002 case-control study conducted by the Centers for Disease Control and Prevention to identify risk factors associated with sporadic *E. coli* O157 infections determined that eating hamburgers cooked in the home was a major risk factor (Kennedy et al., 2002), whereas an earlier case-control study based on data obtained through the same FoodNet system identified eating hamburgers served at table-service restaurants—but not restaurants of major fast-food chains—as a major risk factor (Kassenborg et al., 1998). **The committee recommends that each location—the home, fast-food restaurants, and the remainder of HRI facilities—where ground beef is cooked be modeled separately.** That would necessitate that data on internal temperatures of cooked ground-beef patties be obtained or estimated for the three general locations. The Risk Characterization chapter in the draft correctly notes that "data on variability in food preparation behavior between consumers (home) and food preparers (HRI) are lacking" (p. 141) but this does not necessarily preclude modeling. The committee notes, for example, that most fast-food restaurants that cook patties from the frozen state would not encounter the wide variation in pretreatment storage conditions that was used in the draft to model cooking of ground beef and that variability in pretreatment storage conditions would more likely occur in ground beef cooked in homes.

Caution should be used in applying to the model the data of Jackson et al. (1996) regarding the mean reduction in *E. coli* O157:H7 in grilled ground-beef patties because some of their results (summarized in the draft's Table 3-20) are counterintuitive. There are several observations where greater or equivalent *E. coli* O157:H7 populations were killed at 62.8°C (145°F) than at 68.3°C (155°F). It is well established that the higher the temperature (above the maximal growth temperature), the greater the number of bacteria killed. Furthermore, pretreatment by freezing may increase the sensitivity of pathogens like *E. coli* O157:H7 to thermal inactivation. The Jackson et al. data contradict that: more *E. coli* O157:H7 were inactivated at equivalent cooking temperatures in patties previously held refrigerated at 3°C for 9 hours than in patties held frozen at 18°C for 8 days. **The committee recommends that, until more reliable data become available, D values[3] established for *E. coli* O157:H7 inactivation in ground beef be used to model the effect of pretreatment storage conditions on rates of *E. coli* O157:H7 inactivation. The analysis should account for the varied fat content of ground beef used in the home, fast-food restaurants, and other HRI environments.**

Estimates of Amount of Raw Ground Beef Consumed Are Flawed

The draft model calculates that "cooking" does not yield any log reduction of *E. coli* O157:H7 in 4–8% of ground beef servings. The explanation—described in a footnote (on p. 89)—is that the USDA's Continuing Survey of Food Intakes by Individuals (CSFII) data used as the sole reference reported that four people (three 25–64 years old and one less than 5 years old) consumed "raw" ground beef. For modeling purposes, the servings were considered to be a subset of servings that had no log reduction in *E. coli* O157:H7 during cooking (for example, grossly undercooked servings). That information is critical to understanding the rationale for the relatively high occurrence of no-log-reduction ground-beef servings. **Because of the importance of log-reduction information for interpreting calculated estimates, the committee recommends that the material in the footnote be moved to the text after the estimates that are presented as having no log reduction.**

More important, simple extrapolation of data from the 1994–1996 and 1998 CSFII surveys for estimating the annual number of raw ground-beef servings is scientifically unfounded because of the small number of obser-

---

[3] D (or *decimal reduction*) *value* is the amount of time in minutes required to reduce the number of organisms of a particular bacterium by 90% at a specified temperature. A 90% reduction—from 10^6 to 10^5 colony-forming units, for example—is equivalent to a 1-log decrease.

vations available in some subsets. Table 3-24 in the draft indicates that children 0–5 years old eat an estimated 522,315 servings of raw ground beef annually away from home but none at home. That calculation is based on a single observation, and confidence intervals are not included. **The committee recommends that FSIS acknowledge that it lacks adequate information on the consumption of raw ground beef in the United States.** Linear scaling of observations from one or a small number of individuals to the entire US population is statistically inappropriate. **The committee believes that in this circumstance expert judgment, with appropriate accounting for uncertainty, may be superior to using extant data and suggests that FSIS solicit such input in the short term.**[4] For the longer term, the committee suggests that **better data on raw-meat consumption be gathered and that research account for the fact that some groups of individuals consume raw ground beef in traditional dishes or in keeping with cultural traditions.** USDA's Agricultural Marketing Service or industry sources may have additional information bearing on this question.

Human Exposure to E. coli *O157:H7 in Ground Beef Fails to Address Potentially Important Variables*

The primary outputs of the FSIS draft Preparation Module are estimates of distributions that describe the prevalence of E. coli O157:H7 in ground-beef servings prepared during the seasons in which E. coli O157:H7 is more and less prevalent in cattle at slaughter. The Preparation Module relies solely on outputs of the Slaughter Module related to seasonal differences rather than using FSIS ground-beef sampling data. In addition, considering the major differences in handling of frozen ground beef and in cooking ground beef between fast-food restaurants and the home, there may be substantial differences in distributions of E. coli O157:H7 in ground-beef servings, depending on the location where the meat is prepared, cooked, and consumed. **The committee recommends that FSIS ground-beef sampling data be used to determine seasonal differences in** E. coli **O157:H7 contamination of ground beef and that inputs into the model be further differentiated on the basis of location of ground-beef preparation and consumption.**

Insight into another potentially important variable is provided by the CSFII. The 1994–1996 data regarding ground-beef consumption, repro-

---

[4] Faced with a similar problem in their risk assessment of Shiga-producing *E. coli* O157 in steak tartare, Dutch researchers convened an expert solicitation workshop to estimate values for parameters for which no data were found (Nauta et al., 2001).

TABLE 4-1 Ground-beef quantity (g) consumed per eating occasion by age and sex (2-day sample)

	Age, years									
	2–5	6–11	12–19		20–39		40–59		60 and above	
	M|F	M|F	M	F	M	F	M	F	M	F
Sample Size	2,109	1,432	696	702	1,543	1,449	1,663	1,694	1,545	1,429
Mean	31	41	66	52	80	52	82	57	73	62
Percentile										
5th	1	1	1	1	3	1	3	2	3	2
10th	1	2	2	2	6	3	7	3	8	12
25th	10	16	28	23	38	22	40	24	36	31
50th	24	34	58	44	71	45	70	48	68	54
75th	42	59	88	77	102	77	110	84	96	87
90th	68	85	131	101	155	102	169	112	125	113
95th	85	104	168	127	194	122	200	129	176	140

Source: Smiciklas-Wright et al., 2002 (based on USDA, 2000).

duced below in Table 4-1, suggests that both sex and age are important in serving size. Age is factored in by the model, but sex is not accounted for in the characterization of the quantity of ground-beef products consumed. The gain in precision from including sex is likely to be small compared with other elements for which data are weak or absent. **The committee suggests that the final risk assessment at least note the possible role of sex for completeness and future reference.**

REFERENCES

Audits International. 1999. Audits International Home Food Safety Survey. http://www.foodriskclearinghouse.umd.edu/audits_international.htm, accessed June 10, 2002.

Audits International. 2001. Audits International 2000 Home Food Safety Study.

Buchanan RL, Doyle MP. 1997. Foodborne disease significance of *Escherichia coli* O157:H7 and other enterohemorrhagic *E. coli*. Food Technology 51:69–75.

CDC (Centers for Disease Control and Prevention). 1996. Outbreak of *Escherichia coli* O157:H7 infection Georgia and Tennessee June 1995. Morbidity and Mortality Weekly Report 45(12):249–251.

FDA (Food and Drug Administration). 2000. Report of the FDA Retail Food Program Database of Foodborne Illness Risk Factors. FDA Retail Food Program Steering Committee. August 10, 2000.

Jackson, TC, Hardin MD, Acuff GR. 1996. Heat resistance of *Escherichia coli* O157:H7 in a nutrient medium and in ground beef patties as influenced by storage and holding temperatures. Journal of Food Protection 59:230–237.

Kassenborg H, Hedberg C, Evans M, Chin G, Fiorentino T, Vugia D, Bardsley M, Slutsker L, Griffin P. 1998. Case-control study of sporadic *Escherichia coli* O157:H7 infections in 5 FoodNet sites. Abstracts of the International Conference on Emerging Infectious Diseases, p. 50.

Kennedy, MH, Rabatsky-Ehr T, Thomas SM, Lance-Parker S, Mohle-Boetani J, Smith K, Keene W, Sparling P, Hardnett FP, Mead PS, and the EIP FoodNet Working Group. 2002. Risk factors for sporadic *Escherichia coli* O157 infections in the United States: A case-control study in FoodNet sites, 1999–2000. Abstracts of the International Conference on Emerging Infectious Diseases, p. 169.

Mead PS, Finelli L, Lambert-Fair MA, Champ D, Townes J, Hutwagner L, Barrett T, Spitalny K, Mintz E. 1997. Risk factors for sporadic infection with *Escherichia coli* O157:H7. Archives of Internal Medicine 157(2):204–208.

Nauta MJ, Evers EG, Takumi K, Havelaar AH. 2001. Risk assessment of Shiga-toxin producing *Escherichia coli* O157 in steak tartare in the Netherlands. Rijksinstituut voor Volksgezondheid en Milieu (RIVM). Report 257851 003.

Smiciklas-Wright H, Mitchell DC, Mickle SJ, Cook AJ, Goldman JD. 2002. Foods Commonly Eaten in the United States: Quantities Consumed per Eating Occasion and in a Day, 1994–1996. US Department of Agriculture NFS Report No. 96-5, prepublication version. http://www.barc.usda.gov/bhnrc/foodsurvey/Products9496.html, accessed July 10, 2002.

USDA (US Department of Agriculture), Agricultural Research Service. 2000. Continuing Survey of Food Intakes by Individuals 1994–96, 1998. National Technical Information Service. CD-ROM. NTIS Accession no. PB2000-500027.

5

Hazard Characterization

The Food Safety and Inspection Service (FSIS) draft risk assessment Hazard Characterization chapter describes a method to estimate the number of symptomatic infections resulting from the consumption of cooked ground beef contaminated with *Escherichia coli* O157:H7. This is considered to be a type of "dose-response assessment." The principal concepts contained in the chapter are these:

- generating an adjusted estimate of the annual disease burden of symptomatic *E. coli* O157:H7 infections that is derived by using FoodNet data and making corrections for underdiagnosis and underreporting;
- estimating the proportion of all *E. coli* O157:H7 cases that are due to ground-beef exposure (ingestion);
- deriving the dose-response function for *E. coli* O157:H7 by using data from three sources: the estimated annual number of symptomatic *E. coli* O157:H7 infections due to ground-beef exposure, the estimated number of contaminated ground-beef servings (from the exposure assessment), and the upper- and lower-bound dose-response curves based on surrogate pathogens; and
- validating the derived dose-response function for *E. coli* O157:H7 by comparison with data from an outbreak associated with ground beef on which clinical, epidemiologic, and bacteriologic (isolation of pathogen from uncooked hamburger patties) data were available.

REVIEW OF THE HAZARD CHARACTERIZATION CHAPTER

The draft's discussions of the baseline number of *E. coli* O157:H7 infections and adjustments for underdiagnosis and underreporting are scientifically sound. The logic followed is clear, and the epidemiologic data are used in a reasonable and plausible way. However, by focusing solely on the O157:H7 serotype of enterohemorrhagic *E. coli* and on direct contamination, the draft underestimates the overall burden of disease caused by this category of pathogen and the benefit that could derive from interventions.

O157:H7 as One Member of the Enterohemorrhagic *E. coli* Category of *E. coli* Pathogen

Strains of the O157:H7 serotype of *Escherichia coli* isolated since the early 1980s typically carry a set of virulence factors encoded by chromosomal, plasmid, and phage genes that allow them to cause a spectrum of clinical illness in humans ranging from watery diarrhea and hemorrhagic colitis to hemolytic uremic syndrome (HUS) and thrombotic thrombocytopenic purpura (TTP). It is the last two severe clinical syndromes, particularly HUS, that make O157:H7 an important public health problem in the United States because they may result in hospitalization, chronic disease, and death.

The virulence properties that allow O157:H7 to cause hemorrhagic colitis, HUS, and TTP are common to a category of diarrheogenic *E. coli* often called enterohemorrhagic *E. coli,* or EHEC. It is important to recognize that a number of serotypes of *E. coli* other than O157:H7 also possess these properties. The common virulence factors carried by EHEC include a chromosomal pathogenicity island that encodes proteins allowing the bacteria to cause attaching and effacing lesions of the intestinal mucosa, an approximately 60 megadalton plasmid that encodes attachment factors and an enterohemolyin, and bacteriophages that encode Shiga toxins 1, 2, or both. That array of virulence properties stably carried by some *E. coli* strains makes them "EHEC" and renders them capable of causing the severe diseases that stimulate the demand for interventions.

It should be emphasized that the vast majority of *E. coli* strains associated with HUS and hemorrhagic colitis carry the full array of virulence traits. Most of, although not all, those strains are in a known set of O:H serotypes of which O157:H7 is the most common. Others include O111:H8, O111:NM, O26:H11, O145:H25, and O103:H21. In contrast, *E. coli* strains that produce only Shiga toxin but do not have other virulence properties are occasionally recovered from stool cultures of healthy people or people with mild diarrhea. Only uncommonly are such strains incriminated in association with HUS.

The Disease Burden of Non-O157:H7 Enterohemorrhagic *E. coli*

O157:H7 is undoubtedly the most common EHEC serotype in the United States and Canada (different *E. coli* serotypes predominate in other parts of the world). Nevertheless, the true prevalence of other EHEC serotypes in the United States and their contribution to the EHEC disease burden have not been well studied. One reason is that most bacteriologic surveillance for EHEC is geared specifically to the detection of O157:H7. Early studies in Canada that incriminated Shiga toxin-producing (referred to at that time as Vero-toxin producing) *E. coli* as a cause of HUS showed an association with multiple serotypes in addition to O157:H7 (Karmali et al., 1985). A nationwide Centers for Disease Control and Prevention study of patients with HUS showed that among pediatric cases, 85% of the patients that yielded EHEC isolates in stool cultures had O157:H7 and 15% had other serotypes (Banatvala et al., 2001). Analyses of several outbreaks of colitis and HUS that used appropriate detection techniques have clearly demonstrated that non-O157:H7 EHEC exists in the United States and is responsible for disease (McCarthy et al., 2001). Moreover, surveillance data from other countries—such as Chile (Cordovez et al., 1992; Ojeda et al., 1995; Prado et al., 1997; Rios et al., 1999), Australia (Elliott et al., 2001), the United Kingdom (Kleanthous et al., 1990), Germany (Beutin et al., 1998; Verweyen et al., 1999), and Italy (Caprioli et al., 1994)—clearly show the importance of EHEC O:H serotypes in addition to O157:H7.

The Hazard Identification chapter of the FSIS draft risk assessment indicates that because *E. coli* O157:H7 is the most important serotype in the United States from a public-health standpoint and because there is a paucity of epidemiologic data on non-O157 serotypes, the risk assessment is limited to *E. coli* O157:H7. The committee acknowledges that decision but points out its implication: whatever risk to US public health the risk assessment attributes to O157:H7 as a ground-beef contaminant, it is an underestimate of the overall risk because other EHEC serotypes also cause disease.

Because non-O157:H7 serotypes contribute to the EHEC disease burden—particularly as a cause of HUS—the committee suggests that the decision to exclude these serotypes be revisited. If the final risk assessment is limited to O157:H7, the committee recommends that the decision and its implications for the model be explicitly discussed in the Hazard Characterization chapter.

Estimating the Number of *E. coli* O157:H7 Illnesses Due to Contaminated Ground Beef (Etiologic Fraction)

The draft's analysis of the etiologic fraction is likely to underestimate the proportion of illness due to ground beef because the only mode of transmission considered is direct consumption (ingestion) of ground beef. However, contaminated raw ground beef may be epidemiologically important and lead to clinical infections even if the meat that is ultimately ingested is properly cooked and harbors no living O157:H7 or other EHEC organisms. The reason is that inadequate cooking, mistakes in food handling, or poor hygiene in the kitchen may lead to cross contamination of other food vehicles that may be eaten raw (salads, for example) or after little heating. Because the inoculum of EHEC necessary to cause disease is believed to be low, such cross contamination may be epidemiologically important (Buchanan and Doyle, 1997). The contribution of this mode of transmission could be diminished by future interventions that decrease the degree of contamination of ground beef. In contrast, interventions that aim to ensure the proper cooking of ground beef would not affect the cases of EHEC that result from compromised handling or hygiene practices and resulting cross contamination.

The committee thus wishes to reiterate the comment offered in its review of the Preparation Module: it suggests that consideration be given to factoring in cross contamination as an additional step. If that is not possible, it recommends that the final risk assessment highlight more clearly the role of cross contamination in *E. coli* O157:H7 infection and emphasize the limitations in the model engendered by a decision to not factor it in.

Deriving the Dose-Response Function for EHEC O157:H7

The *E. coli* O157:H7 dose-response function for the FSIS draft risk assessment was derived by applying data from three sources:

- the estimated annual number of symptomatic *E. coli* O157:H7 infections resulting from ground-beef consumption,
- the estimated annual number of contaminated ground-beef servings, and
- the lower- and upper-bound dose-response curves derived from dose-response data from experimental challenges of volunteers with *Shigella dysenteriae* 1 and enteropathogenic *E. coli* (EPEC).

The first two estimates are generated directly from relevant data. In contrast, in an indirect approach, *S. dysenteriae* 1 and EPEC dose-response data are used to create upper and lower brackets within which the EHEC dose-response relationship is presumed to lie.

Shigella Dose-Response Relationship as Upper Limit of Bracket

The FSIS draft states (p. 115):

> *E. coli* O157:H7 may be most similar to *Shigella* spp. with regard to transmission and infectivity; however, *Shigella* spp. are invasive pathogens that multiply within host epithelial cells, whereas *E. coli* O157:H7 does not. Both are transmitted by food, although humans are the reservoir of *Shigella* spp. contamination of food and water. The probability of infection with low doses of *Shigella* spp. is thought to be high.

Most of those statements are correct. Although *Shigella* may indeed be transmitted by contaminated food and water vehicles, and outbreaks due to contaminated food vehicles have been described, in fact the vast body of accumulated epidemiologic data indicates that *Shigella* are most often transmitted through direct person-to-person contact by means of fecally contaminated hands or fomites.[1] Thus, transmission of *Shigella* correlates with the level of personal hygiene rather than sanitation or food hygiene. Populations that manifest compromised personal hygiene are at high risk of transmission of *Shigella* even in industrialized countries. That explains why *Shigella* (particularly *S. sonnei*) poses a health problem in day-care centers and in custodial institutions that house mentally impaired or psychotic patients.

Most outbreaks of shigellosis exhibit a protracted epidemiologic curve characteristic of person-to-person propagation rather than the abrupt pattern characteristic of point-source food-vehicle contamination. *S. dysenteriae* 1—the Shiga bacillus—is unique among the roughly 40 *Shigella* serotypes and subtypes because of the severity of clinical disease that it causes, including HUS as an uncommon complication (Khin et al., 1987; Raghupathy et al., 1978; Rahaman and Greenough, 1978); its elaboration of Shiga toxin 1 (Keusch et al., 1982; Strockbine et al., 1988); and its ability to cause pandemics that extend for years over wide geographic areas (Gangarosa et al., 1970; Mata et al., 1970; Rahaman et al., 1975). The main mode of transmission during Shiga dysentery pandemics is person-to-person spread (Ebright et al., 1984; Gangarosa et al., 1970).

Those epidemiologic observations suggest that minute inocula are capable of causing shigellosis and that *Shigella* may be relatively resistant

---

[1] A fomite is any inanimate object via which pathogenic organisms may be transferred (a knife, for example). A fomite does not support the growth of the pathogen.

to the effects of the gastric acid barrier that constitutes a potent defense against many other bacterial enteropathogens. Many other bacterial enteropathogens require relatively large inocula to cause clinical illness and typically require transmission via food vehicles to allow them to pass through the gastric barrier. Results of volunteer studies with multiple *Shigella* serotypes show that small inocula can cause notable attack rates (DuPont et al., 1989). Moreover, *Shigella* can cause diarrheal illness in volunteers when administered without a buffer like $NaHCO_3$ (which neutralizes gastric acid). Older data are available from volunteer studies with *S. dysenteriae* 1 and *S. flexneri* 2a, whereas more recent dose-response data on experimental challenges with *S. sonnei* and *S. flexneri* 2a are available. The most extensive recent data come from challenges with *S. flexneri* 2a. Although *Shigella* species administered without buffer can cause diarrheal illness, administering *Shigella* in 150 ml of water containing 2.0 grams of $NaHCO_3$ buffer results in higher attack rates and a more consistent clinical illness pattern (discussed further below).

Accumulated epidemiologic data show that EHEC O157:H7 is most often transmitted by ingestion of a contaminated food vehicle (Griffin and Tauxe, 1991). Nevertheless, EHEC can, like *Shigella*, be transmitted directly person to person, particularly in young children and in the elderly (Carter et al., 1987; Ostroff et al., 1990; Pavia et al., 1990; Spika et al., 1986). Thus, as in the case of *Shigella*, there are reports of transmission of EHEC by direct contact within day-care centers and institutions for the elderly. In vitro studies show that EHEC (Duffy et al., 2000; Koodie and Dhople, 2001; Lin et al., 1996), like *Shigella* (Gorden and Small, 1993; Small et al., 1994), exhibit an unusual degree of acid resistance among bacterial enteropathogens. The fact that ground beef and some other common food vehicles responsible for transmission of EHEC O157:H7 involve cooking means that the ingested inocula, like those of *Shigella*, can be quite small. However, the fact that the organisms are ingested in a food vehicle undoubtedly offers the surviving EHEC a degree of protection against the gastric defense barrier. It may thus be the case that the most appropriate dose-response data to use from *Shigella* challenges are those involving administration of *Shigella* with buffer.

Taken together, the above comments strongly support the relevance of the decision to use dose-response data from *Shigella* for the upper limit of the bracket. The data further argue that the EHEC dose-response function is likely to be *very close* to that of *Shigella*.[2] Arguably, it may

---

[2] The draft report does note, on p. 119, that the dose-response function "more clearly approximates that estimated for *Shigella dysenteriae* than for EPEC."

be most appropriate to use dose-response data from experimental challenges with *Shigella* administered with buffer.

Vehicle of Transmission and Mode of Ingestion Affect the Dose-Response Curve of Bacterial Enteropathogens

In attempting to derive a dose-response function for EHEC by using dose-response data from other bacterial enteropathogens, such as *Shigella* and EPEC, the draft's authors focus only on dose. They do not address the precise context in which the dose (inoculum) is ingested. In fact, such context is fundamental when considering the epidemiologic relevance of dose-response data. That is best illustrated by using dose-response data from *Vibrio cholerae* O1, because this example constitutes an extreme. Consider the following observations:

- When fasting healthy adult US volunteers ingested 10^6 colony-forming units (CFU) of *V. cholerae* O1 suspended in water without either buffer or food, neither infection nor diarrhea ensued (Cash et al., 1974; Levine et al., 1981).
- When fasting healthy adult US volunteers ingested 10^6 CFU of *V. cholerae* O1 with $NaHCO_3$ buffer (which neutralizes gastric acid), about 90% became infected and 90% developed cholera diarrhea (Levine et al., 1979a, 1981, 1988; Tacket et al., 1995a).
- When fasting healthy adult US volunteers ingested 10^6 CFU of *V. cholerae* O1 with food (a quasi-Bengali meal), the attack rate for cholera diarrhea (about 90%), the infection rate, and the clinical severity were identical with those observed when the same dose was administered with $NaHCO_3$ buffer (Levine et al., 1981).
- When fasting healthy adult US volunteers were given much lower doses of *V. cholerae* O1 (as low as 10^3 CFU) with $NaHCO_3$ buffer, attack rates for diarrhea remained high (67%), but its severity diminished (Levine et al., 1981).

Those results emphasize that both the dose and the context in which the bacteria are ingested are important determinants of disease. The same dose may be innocuous or cause cholera in 90% of subjects, depending on how the inoculum is ingested. Although the phenomenon is less prominent with some other bacterial enteropathogens, it is nevertheless a factor, even with *Shigella*.

Effect of Mode of Ingestion on *S. Flexneri* 2a Attack Rate

Because the upper bound of the presumed *E. coli* O157:H7 dose-response function that is set by the *S. dysenteriae* 1 data is critical, it is important to examine the data critically. Two constraints can be cited with respect to the *S. dysenteriae* 1 dose-response data that were used to craft an upper limit of the bracket. First, the studies cited in the draft were carried out more than 30 years ago (Levine et al., 1973), and there were some shortcomings in the clinical methods used at that time; in the ensuing decades, methods used in challenge studies have become more rigorous. Second, it is now recognized from challenge studies with *S. flexneri* 2a that the dose-response relationship of *Shigella* can be substantially influenced by how the challenge inoculum is administered to the volunteers in the experimental challenge studies.

Those observations come from multiple challenge studies with *S. flexneri* 2a that involve challenge inocula prepared by the same laboratory (the Center for Vaccine Development of the University of Maryland School of Medicine). Clinical supervision of the studies that generated eight of the nine datasets was provided by one institution (the Center for Vaccine Development; the Walter Reed Army Institute of Research provided clinical supervision of the remaining trial). Five challenge studies were carried out in which inocula containing 10^3 CFU of *S. flexneri* 2a were fed in 45 ml of skim milk to immunologically naive healthy adult community volunteers; the overall clinical attack rate was 48% (24 of 50), with a range of 33% to 58% for attack rates in individual challenge studies. In contrast, three challenges were undertaken in which 10^3 CFU suspended in 150 ml of water containing 2.0 gram of $NaHCO_3$ (to neutralize gastric acid) were fed to groups of immunologically naive volunteers; these three challenges resulted in an overall attack rate of 88% (29 of 33), with individual study attack rates of 86%, 86%, and 92%. The difference in overall response to the same dose administered by two methods is highly significant ($p < 0.01$). The one challenge study in which volunteers ingested 10^2 CFU with $NaHCO_3$ led to an attack rate of 43% (three of seven)—similar to the attack rate encountered when 10^3 CFU were administered without buffer in 45 ml of skim milk. The results of the clinical trials are summarized in Table 5-1.

The above data clearly demonstrate the effect of mode of administration of a *Shigella* inoculum on clinical response, but only two data points are available to construct the dose-response curve. It is notable that the dose-response curve from modern challenge studies with *S. flexneri* 2a administered with buffer is similar to the *S. dysenteriae* 1 dose-response curve based on the early challenges that administered that serotype without buffer. That suggests that the upper limit of the bracket, as constructed, is valid even though the effect of buffering was not factored in. It is unlikely that EHEC would elicit a higher attack rate than *S. dysenteriae* 1 at the same dose. **The committee suggests that—in order to strengthen**

TABLE 5-1 Attack rates with different doses (CFU) of *S. flexneri* 2a administered without or with buffer

Challenge Inoculum (CFU)	Attack Rate When Administered Without Buffer[a]	Reference	Attack Rate When Administered with Buffer[b]	Reference
10^2			3/7 (43%)	
10^3	58% (7/12)	Kotloff et al., 1992	92% (11/12)	Kotloff et al., 1995a
10^3	33% (3/9)	Kotloff et al., 1992	86% (12/14)	Kotloff et al., 1995b
10^3	45% (5/11)	Tacket et al., 1992	86% (6/7)	Coster et al., 1999
10^3	57% (4/7)	Tacket et al., 1992		
10^3	45% (5/11)	Tacket et al., 1992		

[a] Given in 45 ml of skim milk.
[b] Suspended in 150 ml of water containing 2.0 g of $NaHCO_3$.

the scientific foundation for the decision to use dose-response data for *S. dysenteriae* 1 to construct the upper bracket—the final risk assessment discuss how the mode of ingestion affects expected attack rates.

Extrapolation of Dose-Response Data to High-Risk Age Groups

Whatever dose-response data (from studies with *Shigella* or other bacterial enteropathogens) are used as surrogates to help to estimate the dose-response relationship for O157:H7 and other EHEC, it must be remembered that the data are derived from experimental challenge studies in healthy adults. One must extrapolate the data to assess their relevance to the dose-response relationship for toddlers, preschool children, and the elderly, the age groups that suffer the highest incidence of severe clinical outcomes. For *Shigella*, the dose-response data derived from adults appear to be compatible with epidemiologic patterns of endemic shigellosis in which peak incidence rates are observed in children 1–4 years old. Comparable data for the elderly are lacking.

EPEC Dose-Response as Lower Limit of Bracket

The use of EPEC dose-response data as the lower limit is reasonable but somewhat more problematic than the use of *Shigella* data to set the upper bracket. One argument in favor of using EPEC data is that EPEC, like EHEC, contain the chromosomal locus that encodes genes involved in attaching to and effacing intestinal mucosa. However, epidemiologic data do not support the relevance of this model. Few data incriminate EPEC as a cause of outbreaks of diarrhea in older children or adults (Levine, 1987; Levine and Edelman, 1984). Rather, in the wild, EPEC are pathogenic in very young infants. Indeed, in developing countries, the pathogen can be incriminated only within the first 6 months of life, when a substantially higher rate of isolation of EPEC is found in cases with diarrhea than in nondiarrheal controls (Levine et al., 1993). Beyond that age group, the isolation rates are equal.

When EPEC are fed to adult volunteers, moderate to high attack rates of diarrheal illness ensue (Bieber et al., 1998; Donnenberg et al., 1993; Levine et al., 1978). However, the inocula required tend to be rather large $\geq 10^8$ logs) and the bacteria must be fed with buffer to protect them from gastric acid (Levine et al., 1978). Moreover, the incubation period is extraordinarily short, and the diarrheal illness tends to be short-lived (although severe cholera-like purging was induced by one strain at high dosage) (Levine et al., 1978). EPEC is indeed likely to be less pathogenic than EHEC with respect to the inoculum required to induce a clinical response. However, EPEC challenge of adults is an artificial system not usually found in nature.

Role of Host Factors in Clinical Response to Challenge with Bacterial Enteropathogens

It is obvious in experimental challenge studies that different healthy adults may respond differently to ingestion of identical inocula of a bacterial enteropathogen. Prior immunity or nonspecific innate immune mechanisms can partly explain the differences. However, other host factors that represent genetic susceptibilities (or protective factors) may also play an important role in the clinical response. The extreme susceptibility of persons of blood group O to cholera gravis and the role of diminished gastric acid production in the development of severe cholera are examples (Levine et al., 1979b; Nalin et al., 1978; Tacket et al., 1995b).

Dose-Response Curves of Other Possible Bacterial Enteropathogens That Might Serve as Alternatives to Set Lower Limit of Bracket

Dose-response studies of other bacterial enteropathogens have been carried out in healthy volunteers, including enterotoxigenic *E. coli* (ETEC), enteroinvasive *E. coli* (EIEC), enteroaggregative *E. coli* (EAggEC), diffusely adherent *E. coli* (DAEC), *Campylobacter jejuni*, *Salmonella enterica* serovar Typhi, and *V. cholerae* O1, O139, and non-O1/non-O139. Some of these fall in between the dose-response of *Shigella* and EPEC and, arguably, might serve as a more rational source for a lower limit to bracket the presumed EHEC dose-response relationship. Table 5-2 summarizes epidemiologic, pathogenetic, and clinical characteristics of the enteropathogens.

The committee believes that the EPEC dose-response relationship is a conservative choice for the lower limit and suggests that—if the bounding approach continues to be used in the final risk assessment—consideration be given to alternatives like these that might reflect the pathogenicity of EHEC better.

Uncertainty in Cases and Exposure Distribution

The FSIS draft risk assessment properly notes that "uncertainty about the *E. coli* O157:H7 dose-response function extends almost across the full range enveloped by the lower and upper bound curves" (p. 119). This is an important statement and is likely to be correct for all the reasons mentioned in the other comments. Overall, the draft chapter's authors did an elegant job in generating an EHEC dose-response function. According to

TABLE 5-2 Epidemiologic, pathogenetic, and clinical characteristics of EHEC-like enteropathogens

Pathogen	Reservoir	Foodborne?	Epithelial-Cell Invasiveness?	Natural Pathogen for Adults and Children?	References
ETEC (human)	Humans	Yes	No	Yes	DuPont et al., 1971; Levine et al., 1977; Levine et al., 1979c
EIEC	Humans	Yes	Yes	Yes	DuPont et al., 1971
EAggEC	Humans	?	No	?	Nataro et al., 1995
DAEC	?	?	No	?	Tacket et al., 1990
C. jejuni	Animals	Yes	Yes	Yes	Black et al., 1988
S. Typhi	Humans	Yes	Yes	Yes	Hornick et al., 1970
V. cholerae O1	Environment	Yes (seafood; water)	No	Yes	Levine et al., 1981; Levine et al., 1979b
V. cholerae O139	Environment	Yes	No	Yes	Tacket et al., 1995a
V. cholerae non-O1/non-O139	Environment	Yes (seafood)	Some	Yes	Morris et al., 1990

Figure 4-5 of the draft, the 50th percentile derived dose-response curve predicts an ingested dose of ~4.8 logs (~63,000 organisms) of EHEC will result in clinical illness in 50% of subjects. The dose of *S. dysenteriae* 1 that is expected to cause a 50% attack rate is ~2.9 logs (~740 organisms). Thus, the FSIS draft model suggests that the dose-response curve for EHEC is somewhat to the right of that of *Shigella* (requires more organisms). This model suggests that up to 2 logs more EHEC must be ingested to result in the same attack rate as *Shigella*.

Severe Clinical Outcomes and Sensitive Populations

The FSIS draft offers two observations regarding severe clinical outcomes and sensitive populations that the committee would like to highlight.

It asserts that "estimating the clinical outcomes of symptomatic infection is essential for future cost-benefit analyses of intervention options" (p. 121). That is an important point. As previously stated, it is the propensity for EHEC to cause severe illness, chronic disease, and death—particularly in young children—that makes it an important public-health problem and stimulates the demand for interventions. Thus, the risk assessment should focus primarily on HUS (for simplicity, TTP may be considered a variant of HUS seen in adults) as a clinical outcome. If O157:H7 and other EHEC caused only gastroenteritis, they would be in the same category, as a public-health problem, as *Campylobacter jejuni* and nontyphoidal *Salmonella enterica* and might well have a less prominent public profile. By extension, it may be strongly argued that whatever interventions are contemplated, both public health authorities and the general public will expect them to significantly diminish the burden of HUS and other serious outcomes.

The draft also notes that "the reason why children have the highest reported incidence of *E. coli* O157:H7 infection is not known" (p. 123). It proceeds to offer several possible explanations, including differences in health-care patterns (health care may be more likely to be sought for children), exposure differences, and biologic differences. The draft offers a fair and honest statement of the lack of data to explain the observed age differences in clinical expression. The lack of data, however, should not be an obstacle to evaluating the disproportionate risk that children—and the elderly (who are omitted from the chapter's discussion of sensitive subpopulations)—manifest for severe clinical outcomes. This issue and the committee's recommendations regarding it are addressed in the review of the draft risk characterization—the next chapter of this review.

Validation of E. coli O157:H7 Dose-Response Function Using Outbreak Data

Using data from a 1992–1993 hamburger-associated outbreak that included clinical, epidemiologic, and microbiologic information, an analysis presented in the FSIS draft estimates that the 45-gram contaminated hamburgers consumed during the outbreak harbored a median of about 96 CFU of *E. coli* O157:H7 before cooking. That is similar to the data of Tuttle et al. (1999), who calculated that the median dose of O157:H7 in hamburger patties associated with a large outbreak was 67.5 CFU before cooking. Assuming that even inadequate cooking results in a diminution of the inoculum, the dose ingested must indeed be quite small. Although not mentioned in the text, this is further evidence that the dose required to cause EHEC disease is similar to the low doses of *Shigella* that can cause disease. The concentration of pediatric cases in the outbreak also underscores the importance of focusing attention on this population in the risk characterization.

SUMMARY REMARKS

Overall, the FSIS draft risk assessment's authors did an excellent job with the hazard characterization, given the limitations of data and gaps in data. Their model is elegant, and they use a logical progression of steps in this chapter. One might argue with the use of EPEC dose-response data to serve as the lower limit of a presumed EHEC dose-response function. In fact, epidemiologic and microbiologic data suggest that the true EHEC dose-response function is likely to resemble that of *Shigella*.

The failure to account for non-O157:H7 as a cause of hemorrhagic colitis and HUS underestimates the overall burden of EHEC disease in the United States and the benefits that may derive from future interventions. The true burden of severe EHEC disease probably is 15–20% greater than estimates based on O157:H7 alone.

REFERENCES

Banatvala N, Griffin PM, Greene KD, Barrett TJ, Bibb WF, Green JH, Wells JG. 2001. The United States National Prospective Hemolytic Uremic Syndrome Study: Microbiologic, serologic, clinical, and epidemiologic findings. Journal of Infectious Diseases 183:1063–1070.

Beutin L, Zimmermann S, Gleier K. 1998. Human infections with Shiga toxin-producing *Escherichia coli* other than serogroup O157 in Germany. Emerging Infectious Diseases 4:635–639.

Bieber D, Ramer SW, Wu CY, Murray WJ, Tobe T, Fernandez R, Schoolnik GK. 1998. Type IV pili, transient bacterial aggregates, and virulence of enteropathogenic *Escherichia coli*. Science 280:2114–2118.

Buchanan RL, Doyle MP. 1997. Foodborne disease significance of *Escherichia coli* O157:H7 and other enterohemorrhagic *E. coli*. Food Technology 51:69–75.

Black RE, Levine MM, Clements ML, Hughes TP, Blaser MJ. 1988. Experimental *Campylobacter jejuni* infection in humans. Journal of Infectious Diseases 157:472–479.
Caprioli A, Luzzi I, Rosmini F, Resti C, Edefonti A, Perfumo F, Farina C, Goglio A, Gianviti A, Rizzoni G. 1994. Community-wide outbreak of hemolytic-uremic syndrome associated with non-O157 verocytotoxin-producing *Escherichia coli*. Journal of Infectious Diseases 169:208–211.
Carter AO, Borczyk AA, Carlson JA, Harvey B, Hockin JC, Karmali MA, Krishnan C, Korn DA, Lior H. 1987. A severe outbreak of *Escherichia coli* O157:H7-associated hemorrhagic colitis in a nursing home. New England Journal of Medicine 317:1496–1500.
Cash RA, Music SI, Libonati JP, Snyder MJ, Wenzel RP, Hornick RB. 1974. Response of man to infection with *Vibrio cholerae*. I. Clinical, serologic, and bacteriologic responses to a known inoculum. Journal of Infectious Diseases 129:45–52.
Cordovez A, Prado V, Maggi L, Cordero J, Martinez J, Misraji A, Rios R, Soza G, Ojeda A, Levine MM. 1992. Enterohemorrhagic *Escherichia coli* associated with hemolytic-uremic syndrome in Chilean children. Journal of Clinical Microbiology 30:2153–2157.
Coster TS, Hoge CW, VanDeVerg LL, Hartman AB, Oaks EV, Venkatesan MM, Cohen D, Robin G, Fontaine-Thompson A, Sansonetti PJ, Hale TL. 1999. Vaccination against shigellosis with attenuated *Shigella flexneri* 2a strain SC602. Infection and Immunity 67:3437–3443.
Donnenberg MS, Tacket CO, James SP, Losonsky G, Nataro JP, Wasserman SS, Kaper JB, Levine MM. 1993. Role of the eaeA gene in experimental enteropathogenic Escherichia coli infection. Journal of Clinical Investigation 92:1412–1417.
Duffy LL, Grau FH, Vanderlinde PB. 2000. Acid resistance of enterohaemorrhagic and generic *Escherichia coli* associated with foodborne disease and meat. International Journal of Food Microbiology 60:83–89.
DuPont HL, Formal SB, Hornick RB, Snyder MJ, Libonati JP, Sheahan DG, LaBrec EH, Kalas JP. 1971. Pathogenesis of *Escherichia coli* diarrhea. New England Journal of Medicine 285: 1–9.
DuPont HL, Levine MM, Hornick RB, Formal SB. 1989. Inoculum size in shigellosis and implications for expected mode of transmission. Journal of Infectious Diseases 159:1126–1128.
Ebright JR, Moore EC, Sanborn WR, Schaberg D, Kyle J, Ishida K. 1984. Epidemic Shiga bacillus dysentery in Central Africa. American Journal of Tropical Medicine and Hygiene 33:1192–1197.
Elliott EJ, Robins-Browne RM, O'Loughlin EV, Bennett-Wood V, Bourke J, Henning P, Hogg GG, Knight J, Powell H, Redmond D. 2001. Nationwide study of haemolytic uraemic syndrome: Clinical, microbiological, and epidemiological features. Archives of Disease in Childhood 85:125–131.
Gangarosa EJ, Perera DR, Mata LJ, Mendizabal-Morris C, Guzman G, Reller LB. 1970. Epidemic Shiga bacillus dysentery in Central America. II. Epidemiologic studies in 1969. Journal of Infectious Diseases 122:181–190.
Gorden J, Small PLC. 1993. Acid resistance in enteric bacteria. Infection and Immunity 61:364–367.
Griffin PM, Tauxe RV. 1991. The epidemiology of infections caused by *Escherichia coli* O157:H7, other enterohemorrhagic *E. coli*, and the associated hemolytic uremic syndrome. Epidemiologic Reviews 13:60–98.
Hornick RB, Greisman SE, Woodward TE, DuPont HL, Dawkins AT, Snyder MJ. 1970. Typhoid fever; pathogenesis and immunologic control. New England Journal of Medicine 283:686–691, 739–746.

Karmali MA, Petric M, Lim C, Fleming PC, Arbus GS, Lior H. 1985. The association between idiopathic hemolytic uremic syndrome and infection by verotoxin-producing *Escherichia coli*. Journal of Infectious Diseases 151:775–782.

Keusch GT, Donohue-Rolfe A, Jacewicz M. 1982. *Shigella* toxin(s): Description and role in diarrhea and dysentery. Pharmacology & Therapeutics 15:403–438.

Khin MU, Myo K, Tin A, Myo MA, Soe SA, Thane-Oke KM, Khin TN. 1987. Clinical features, including haemolytic-uraemic syndrome, in *Shigella dysenteriae* type 1 infection in children of Rangoon. Journal of Diarrhoeal Diseases Research 5:175–177.

Kleanthous H, Smith HR, Scotland SM, Gross RJ, Rowe B, Taylor CM, Milford DV. 1990. Haemolytic uraemic syndromes in the British Isles, 1985-8: Association with verocytotoxin producing *Escherichia coli*. Part 2: Microbiological aspects. Archives of Disease in Childhood 65:722–727.

Koodie L, Dhople AM. 2001. Acid tolerance of *Escherichia coli* O157:H7 and its survival in apple juice. Microbios 104:167–175.

Kotloff KL, Herrington DA, Hale TL, Newland JW, Van de Verg L, Cogan JP, Snoy PJ, Sadoff JC, Formal SB, Levine MM. 1992. Safety, immunogenicity, and efficacy in monkeys and humans of invasive *Escherichia coli* K-12 hybrid vaccine candidates expressing *Shigella flexneri* 2a somatic antigen. Infection and Immunity 60:2218–2224.

Kotloff KL, Losonsky GA, Nataro JP, Wasserman SS, Hale TL, Taylor DN, Newland JW, Sadoff JC, Formal SB, Levine MM. 1995a. Evaluation of the safety, immunogenicity and efficacy in healthy adults of four doses of live oral hybrid *Escherichia coli-Shigella flexneri* 2a vaccine strain EcSf2a-2. Vaccine 13:495–502.

Kotloff KL, Nataro JP, Losonsky GA, Wasserman SS, Hale TL, Taylor DN, Sadoff JC, Levine MM. 1995b. A modified *Shigella* volunteer challenge model in which the inoculum is administered with bicarbonate buffer: Clinical experience and implications for *Shigella* infectivity. Vaccine 13:1488–1494.

Levine MM. 1987. *Escherichia coli* that cause diarrhea: enterotoxigenic, enteropathogenic, enteroinvasive, enterohemorrhagic, and enteroadherent. Journal of Infectious Diseases 155:377–389.

Levine MM, Edelman R. 1984. Enteropathogenic *Escherichia coli* of classic serotypes associated with infant diarrhea: epidemiology and pathogenesis. Epidemiologic Reviews 6:31–51.

Levine MM, Dupont HL, Formal SB, Hornick RB, Takeuchi A, Gangarosa EJ, Snyder MJ, Libonati JP. 1973. Pathogenesis of *Shigella dysenteriae* 1 (Shiga) dysentery. Journal of Infectious Diseases 127(3):261–270.

Levine MM, Caplan ES, Waterman D, Cash RA, Hornick RB, Snyder MJ. 1977. Diarrhea caused by *Escherichia coli* that produce only heat-stable enterotoxin. Infection and Immunity 17:78–82.

Levine MM, Bergquist EJ, Nalin DR, Waterman DH, Hornick RB, Young CR, Sotman S, Rowe B. 1978. *Escherichia coli* strains that cause diarrhoea but do not produce heat-labile or heat-stable enterotoxins and are non-invasive. Lancet 1:1119–1122.

Levine MM, Nalin DR, Craig JP, Hoover D, Bergquist EJ, Waterman D, Holley HP, Hornick RB, Pierce NP, Libonati JP. 1979a. Immunity of cholera in man: Relative role of antibacterial versus antitoxic immunity. Transactions of the Royal Society of Tropical Medicine and Hygiene 73:3–9.

Levine MM, Nalin DR, Rennels MB, Hornick RB, Sotman S, Van Blerk G, Hughes TP, O'Donnell S, Barua D. 1979b. Genetic susceptibility to cholera. Annals of Human Biology 6(4):369–374.

Levine MM, Nalin DR, Hoover DL, Bergquist EJ, Hornick RB, Young CR. 1979c. Immunity to enterotoxigenic *Escherichia coli*. Infection and Immunity 23:729–736.

Levine MM, Black RE, Clements ML, Nalin DR, Cisneros L, Finkelstein RA. 1981. Volunteer studies in development of vaccines against cholera and enterotoxigenic *Escherichia coli*: A review. In: Holme T, Holmgren J, Merson MH, Mollby R, eds. Acute Enteric Infections in Children: New Prospects for Treatment and Prevention. Amsterdam: Elsevier/North-Holland Biomedical Press, pp. 443–459.

Levine MM, Kaper JB, Herrington D, Ketley J, Losonsky G, Tacket CO, Tall B, Cryz S. 1988. Safety, immunogenicity, and efficacy of recombinant live oral cholera vaccines, CVD 103 and CVD 103-HgR. Lancet 2:467–470.

Levine MM, Ferreccio C, Prado V, Cayazzo M, Abrego P, Martinez J, Maggi L, Baldini M, Martin W, Maneval D, Kay B, Guers L, Lior H, Wasserman SS, Nataro JP. 1993. Epidemiologic studies of *Escherichia coli* infections in a low socioeconomic level periurban community in Santiago, Chile. American Journal of Epidemiology 138:849–869.

Lin J, Smith MP, Chapin KC, Baik HS, Bennett GN, Foster JW. 1996. Mechanisms of acid resistance in enterohemorrhagic *Escherichia coli*. Applied and Environmental Microbiology 62:3094–3100.

Mata L, Gangarosa E, Caceres A, Perera D, Mejicanos M. 1970. Epidemic *Shiga bacilllus* dysentery in Central America. I. Etiologic investigations in Guatemala, 1969. Journal of Infectious Diseases 122:170–180.

McCarthy TA, Barrett NL, Hadler JL, Salsbury B, Howard RT, Dingman DW, Brinkman CD, Bibb WF, Cartter ML. 2001. Hemolytic-uremic syndrome and *Escherichia coli* O121 at a lake in Connecticut, 1999. Pediatrics 108:E59.

Morris JG Jr, Takeda T, Tall BD, Losonsky GA, Bhattacharya SK, Forrest BD, Kay BA, Nishibuchi M. 1990. Experimental non-01 group1 Vibrio cholerae gastroenteritis in humans. Journal of Clinical Investigation 85:697–705.

Nalin DR, Levine RJ, Levine MM, Hoover D, Bergquist E, McLaughlin J, Libonati J, Alam J, Hornick RB. 1978. Cholera, non-vibrio cholera, and stomach acid. Lancet 2:856–859.

Nataro JP, Deng Y, Cookson S, Cravioto A, Savarino SJ, Guers LD, Levine MM, Tacket CO. 1995. Heterogeneity of enteroaggregative *Escherichia coli* virulence demonstrated in volunteers. Journal of Infectious Diseases 171:465–468.

Ojeda A, Prado V, Martinez J, Arellano C, Borczyk A, Johnson W, Lior H, Levine MM. 1995. Sorbitol-negative phenotype among enterohemorrhagic Escherichia coli strains of different serotypes and from different sources. Journal of Clinical Microbiology 33:2199–2201.

Ostroff SM, Griffin PM, Tauxe RV, Shipman LD, Greene KD, Wells JG, Lewis JH, Blake PA, Kobayashi JM. 1990. A statewide outbreak of *Escherichia coli* O157:H7 infections in Washington State. American Journal of Epidemiology 132:239–247.

Pavia AT, Nichols CR, Green DP, Tauxe RV, Mottice S, Greene KD, Wells JG, Siegler RL, Brewer ED, Hannon D. 1990. Hemolytic-uremic syndrome during an outbreak of *Escherichia coli* O157:H7 infections in institutions for mentally retarded persons: Clinical and epidemiologic observations. Jornal de Pediatria 116:544–551.

Prado V, Martinez J, Arellano C, Levine MM. 1997. [Temporal variation of genotypes and serotypes of enterohemorrhagic *E. coli* isolated from Chilean children with intestinal infections or hemolytic uremic syndrome]. Revista Medica de Chile 125:291–297.

Raghupathy P, Date A, Shastry JC, Sudarsanam A, Jadhav M. 1978. Haemolytic-uraemic syndrome complicating *Shigella* dysentery in south Indian children. British Medical Journal 1(6126):1518–1521.

Rahaman MM, Greenough WB III. 1978. Shigellosis and haemolytic uraemic syndrome. Lancet 1(8072):1051.

Rahaman MM, Khan MM, Aziz KMS, Islam MS, Kibriya AK. 1975. An outbreak of dysentery caused by *Shigella dysenteriae* type 1 on a Coral Island in the Bay of Bengal. Journal of Infectious Diseases 132(1):15–19.

Rios M, Prado V, Trucksis M, Arellano C, Borie C, Alexandre M, Fica A, Levine MM. 1999. Clonal diversity of Chilean isolates of enterohemorrhagic *Escherichia coli* from patients with hemolytic-uremic syndrome, asymptomatic subjects, animal reservoirs, and food products. Journal of Clinical Microbiology 37:778–781.

Small P, Blankenhorn D, Welty D, Zinser E, Slonczewski JL. 1994. Acid and base resistance in *Escherichia coli* and *Shigella flexneri*: Role of rpoS and growth pH. Journal of Bacteriology 176:1729–1737.

Spika JS, Parsons JE, Nordenberg D, Wells JG, Gunn RA, Blake PA. 1986. Hemolytic uremic syndrome and diarrhea associated with *Escherichia coli* O157:H7 in a day care center. Jornal de Pediatria 109:287–291.

Strockbine NA, Jackson MP, Sung LM, Holmes RK, O'Brien AD. 1988. Cloning and sequencing of the genes for Shiga toxin from *Shigella dysenteriae* type 1. Journal of Bacteriology 170:1116–1122.

Tacket CO, Moseley SL, Kay B, Losonsky G, Levine MM. 1990. Challenge studies in volunteers using *Escherichia coli* strains with diffuse adherence to HEp-2 cells. Journal of Infectious Diseases 162:550–552.

Tacket CO, Binion SB, Bostwick E, Losonsky GA, Roy MJ, Edelman R. 1992. Efficacy of bovine milk immunoglobulin concentrate in preventing illness after *Shigella flexneri* challenge. American Journal of Tropical Medicine and Hygiene 47:276–283.

Tacket CO, Losonsky G, Nataro JP, Comstock L, Michalski J, Edelman R, Kaper JB, Levine MM. 1995a. Initial clinical studies of CVD 112 *Vibrio cholerae* O139 live oral vaccine: safety and efficacy against experimental challenge. Journal of Infectious Diseases 172:883–886.

Tacket CO, Losonsky G, Nataro JP, Wasserman SS, Cryz SJ, Edelman R, Levine MM. 1995b. Extension of the volunteer challenge model to study South American cholera in a population of volunteers predominantly with blood group antigen O. Transactions of the Royal Society of Tropical Medicine and Hygiene 89:75–77.

Tuttle J, Gomez T, Doyle MP, Wells JG, Zhao T, Tauxe RV, Griffin PM. 1999. Lessons from a large outbreak of *Escherichia coli* O157:H7 infections: Insights into the infectious dose and method of widespread contamination of hamburger patties. Epidemiology and Infection 122:185–192.

Verweyen HM, Karch H, Allerberger F, Zimmerhackl LB. 1999. Enterohemorrhagic *Escherichia coli* (EHEC) in pediatric hemolytic-uremic syndrome: A prospective study in Germany and Austria. Infection 27:341–347.

6

Risk Characterization

The Risk Characterization chapter of the Food Safety and Inspection Service (FSIS) draft risk assessment integrates and applies the modeling work done in the three modules of the exposure assessment (Production, Slaughter, and Preparation) and the dose-response assessment presented in "Hazard Characterization." The analyses characterize the risk associated with *E. coli* O157:H7 exposure of individuals, the community, and the population for different exposure periods. The effect of seasonal variations in exposure, and therefore risk, is examined with differences in risk to young children. The results of some sample sensitivity analyses are also presented to demonstrate potential policy applications of the model.

In the discussion below, the committee offers observations, suggestions, and recommendations related to the major sections of the draft chapter. Many of the important points it wishes to make have already been addressed in the previous chapters or are more appropriately discussed in the Modeling Approach and Implementation chapter that follows, so this chapter is brief.

DEFINITION OF KEY TERMS

The chapter's definitions are clearly spelled out and helpful in interpreting the material. However, as mentioned elsewhere in this review, some of the draft report's definitions are not the standard ones used in the scientific literature or other quantitative risk assessments. Others include terminology that may confuse readers. Because microbial risk assessment is a relatively new field, it is desirable to promote consistency and clarity in expression. We present below a number of specific suggestions regarding defined and undefined terms.

"Typical" individual risk is the term applied to the risk posed for someone who purchases ground beef that is contaminated with *E. coli* O157:H7 organisms at the median concentration, who stores and cooks that product in a way that is consistent with the median growth and cooking distributions, and who consumes a single serving. Because the definition does not describe a "typical" exposure, the committee suggests that that word be changed, perhaps to *hypothetical* or *illustrative*.

Duration of exposure is defined in the draft as "the length of time (e.g., per serving, per annum, or lifetime) for which a risk estimate was assessed." The definition is confusing. Relating a serving to a *duration* of exposure is awkward. The committee suggests that this term, which is used only twice in text, be dropped.

The term *dose* is defined as the number of *E. coli* O157:H7 in a single serving of ground beef. That is consistent with the draft Food and Drug Administration (FDA)-USDA *Listeria* risk assessment (2001). However, in chemical risk assessments, dose is usually defined as grams per kilogram of body weight of a subject. The committee suggests that the report's definition of *dose* draw attention to the different meaning of this term in microbial risk assessments.

The draft cites *sensitivity analysis* as "the quantitative process of identifying factors (model inputs) in the farm-to-table continuum that contribute to the occurrence of *E. coli* O157:H7 in ground beef or the subsequent risk of illness" (p. 130). That definition is tangentially related to the more traditional understanding of the term: the quantification of the effects of *changes in* model inputs on model outputs. However, it fails to capture the sense in which most risk analysts apply it: the systematic investigation of whether and to what extent changes in model inputs across a plausible range of values affect model outputs. The committee suggests that the final risk assessment adopt the more common definition of *sensitivity analysis*. The related terms *correlation analysis* and *dependency analysis* should also be more clearly and completely documented on the basis of established definitions.

The "risk of illness" is addressed throughout the chapter, but no formal definition of the conditions covered by *illness* is provided. As the draft notes (pp. 22–23), ingestion of *E. coli* O157:H7 can result in a wide array of outcomes, including asymptomatic infection, abdominal cramps, nonbloody diarrhea, hemorrhagic colitis, hemolytic uremic syndrome (HUS), and thrombotic thrombocytopenic purpura (TTP). The chapter needs a clear definition, and, depending on the conditions covered, *risk of infection* may be a more appropriate term. Furthermore, "annual risk" and "risk per serving" are both referred to as *risk of illness* in the chapter. The committee suggests that the text clearly state what is being reported in each instance and, if necessary, use different terms for these metrics to minimize confusion.

In later sections of the chapter, the risk of "severe illness" is evaluated. The term is not defined, although the text (p. 135) refers to hemorrhagic colitis (called "bloody diarrhea"), HUS, and death. The draft's Hazard Characterization chapter lists hospitalization, HUS, TTP, and death in a discussion of "severe clinical outcomes" (p. 121). The committee suggests that the terminology be standardized in the risk assessment and that appropriate definitions be added to this and other sections.

In general, the committee suggests that—where possible—the final risk assessment adopt the definitions established by one of the major organizations that have already published glossaries and that alternative expressions be used in other circumstances. The World Health Organization (WHO, 1995), Codex Alimentarius Commission (1999), and International Life Sciences Institute (ILSI, 2000) have developed sets of definitions that are potential starting points for aligning terminology. The draft FDA-USDA *Listeria* risk assessment (2001) also contains a well-written extended glossary. The committee recognizes that not all terms can be aligned, but it believes that in many cases it would be less confusing if terms were used in a standard way.

The committee also suggests that all the terms in this section and the rest of the draft be provided with general definitions before they are applied specifically to the O157:H7 risk assessment, as is done for the draft's definition of *risk*.

RISK OF ILLNESS FROM *E. COLI* O157:H7

The term *risk of illness* is used in this section to describe the probability of illness from consuming ground beef with different doses of O157:H7. That risk is estimated as the product of the probability of exposure and the probability of illness associated with a given dose. The committee is concerned that the results of this analysis, as presented in the tables and figures in the draft, may be misunderstood by some lay readers. Because the probability of exposure to very large numbers of organisms is relatively small, the risk of illness from such exposure is concomitantly small. The committee is concerned that some may interpret the presentation to mean that the model predicts that one is less likely to become ill from massive doses of *E. coli* O157:H7 than from much smaller exposures. **The committee recommends that these analyses, if retained in the final risk assessment, be expressed as a cumulative probability of illness, given the projected frequency and levels of contamination of ground beef.**

The committee also observes that it would be helpful if a discussion were added to this section that clearly indicates how the modeling of infection differs from the modeling of illness.

Risk of Illness for an Individual

In this subsection, per-serving, annual, and lifetime risks are provided for a "typical" person, on the basis of the point estimates of the model's outputs and the median of the derived dose-response relationship. As noted above, this is in reality a hypothetical person with *an exposure scenario* that could be considered illustrative.

Table 5-1 in the FSIS draft, which presents the information used in this section, is particularly useful in identifying the location of data used in the assessment. The addition of a side-by-side table that summarizes the individual hypothetical risks (per serving, annual, and lifetime) and the associated assumptions in the "typical" exposure scenario would provide additional clarity and bring home the point that a hypothetical individual risk is being calculated.

More generally, the committee believes that the draft's focus on a "typical" person is—from public health and policy perspectives—misguided. It is desirable to avoid all *E. coli* O157:H7 infections, but attention needs to be centered on the more severe outcomes of infection. That means examining the determinants of high exposure in the general population and any exposure in the subpopulations thought to be most vulnerable to complications: children and the elderly.[1] Although some attempt is made to address the special vulnerabilities of children later in the chapter, the analysis is cursory and does not address whether differences in consumption patterns might affect risk. There is no separate consideration of the elderly in the draft.

The committee recommends that the Risk Characterization chapter be refocused to concentrate on the analysis of severe illnesses associated with *E. coli* O157:H7 infection, the subpopulations known or thought to be most vulnerable to them, and the interventions that might have the greatest effect in preventing them.

---

[1] Although immune-compromised individuals are at a greater risk of disease from exposure to some protozoal enteric pathogens (including *Shigella*), an analogous association has not been recognized between severe enterohemorrhagic *E. coli* disease such as HUS and immuno-compromised human hosts.

Risk of Illness for a Community—Simulated Outbreak

This subsection is intended to provide an example of how the presence of *E. coli* O157:H7 in ground beef might contribute to an outbreak. Like the hypothetical individual risk, this risk characterization is based on a prescribed scenario of exposure—an example of what might happen if contamination occurred and were spread at a community level. The risk metric in this section is *risk per serving,* and the analysis estimates the number of illnesses as a function of assumptions regarding the number of servings consumed by each person, the total number of contaminated servings, and the reduction in contamination from cooking.

This brief "what-if" analysis illustrates how an outbreak might occur and provides interesting outputs. However, the committee believes that it is appropriate to address more time and attention to this scenario in the final risk assessment because of the great public interest in community outbreaks. **At a minimum, the committee suggests that a summary table of assumptions in the community-exposure scenario and calculations of risk be added to improve the clarity of the presentation.** This addition will permit the reader to relate estimates of risk per serving to the number of people who could become ill.

The committee also suggests that the assessment address the conditions in the exposure continuum that are likely to lead to outbreaks. Additional examples that demonstrate the effects of storage, handling, and cooking methods on the potential for an outbreak (for example, an analysis of the effect of improper cooking on the risk of a community outbreak) would be helpful, as would a discussion of how likely the various scenarios are. **And the committee recommends that the risk assessment focus its evaluation of community risk on more severe outcomes and effects on vulnerable subpopulations.**

Risk of Illness for the US Population

This subsection summarizes modeling results that are likely to be used often for public health decision-making, and it evaluates the overall risk of illness, given the population distribution of exposure and the dose-response function. The risk characterization for the US population and, as noted above, selected vulnerable subpopulations should thus be the central output of the risk assessment.

The committee notes that the authors indicate that they will address other populations' risk variability as more data become available. It supports that plan and recommends that additional analyses be presented in the final report based on available data to test the effects of different assumptions and model parameters. The analyses could include estimates of risk associated with different storage and cooking practices.

The statement that the population risk estimate from this report is "comparable" with risks estimated by other investigators (p. 135) is overstated. The estimated 9.6×10^{-7} annual risk of illness in the draft risk assessment is 2 orders of magnitude lower than that reported by Cassin et al. in 1998 (5.1×10^{-5} for adults), and the upper bound of this risk assessment is 3 orders of magnitude lower than the upper bound of Marks and colleagues' in 1998 (10^{-7} versus 10^{-4}). Chapter 7 of the present review provides additional discussion of this point.

The explanation of differences between the number of cases per year from the draft model and that based on surveillance data is incomplete. Attributes of data used in the risk assessment might contribute to the differences; for example, the estimate of ground-beef servings consumed per year could be an underestimate.

Given the anchoring approach used in the draft, the committee questions the informativeness of the estimation of the risk of severe illness presented at the end of the subsection because the model is already adjusted to conform to observed levels of illness. Furthermore, as noted elsewhere, the risk of severe illness is highly age-dependent. Either age dependence should be addressed in this subsection, or the analysis should be dropped. Again, these points are addressed in greater detail in Chapter 7 of this review.

For clarity, the committee suggests that the X axes of Figures 5-1 and 5-2—labeled "Dose"—be relabeled "Number of *E. coli* O157:H7 per Serving" to relate them more directly to the data and analysis summarized in Table 5-2 in the draft risk assessment.

POPULATION RISK BY SEASON, AGE, AND LOCATION

This is an important section, and the authors have clearly noted that. It is less clear whether the appropriate metric has been applied.

Intuition suggests a pronounced seasonal effect in preparation, handling, and consumption of ground beef associated with fair-weather activities, such as outdoor grilling, picnicking, and camping. **The committee suggests that if such seasonal factors can be explicitly addressed, they should be. If data are insufficient to allow their effects to be analyzed, seasonal effects beyond the changes in *E. coli* O157:H7 prevalence now addressed need to be recognized, and the resulting limitations acknowledged.**

As noted above, the analysis of the risks to children is cursory at best, and the special risks to the elderly are not evaluated. If this analysis is to be used to set policy that affects public health, it needs to address the special vulnerabilities of these sections of the population.

The committee agrees that there are likely to be great differences in food-preparation practices between hotels, restaurants, and institutions (HRI) and home environments, and it points out that practices in the fast-food mass-retail establishments—where a considerable proportion of ground-beef meals are prepared and consumed—may differ from those of other HRI businesses. The draft risk assessment correctly notes this as a research need. HRI businesses and trade associations may well already have the information needed to allow analysis of the issue, and the committee recommends that their input be solicited.

SENSITIVITY ANALYSIS

Sensitivity analysis is an important aspect of a risk characterization. **The committee recommends that a discussion of the types of analyses that are available within the Risk Characterization Module and a rationale for the selection of the most appropriate analysis for a given situation be included.** In the case of correlation analysis, the degree of uncertainty in the model inputs should be clearly stated, in addition to the presentation of the correlation outputs.

The dependence analysis presented in this section appears to arbitrarily introduce a 50% change in the model input's assumptions (that is, feedlot prevalence, steam pasteurization, and the like). If there is any rationale for the new assumptions, it should be stated. Otherwise, it should be made clear that they are being presented for illustrative purposes only.

On p. 149 of the draft, preparation scenarios 2 and 3 are based on cooking to 5-log reduction. The reader would benefit from an explanation of the motivation for picking this level of reduction, given that the draft report indicates (in a footnote on p. 131) that a 5.5-log reduction is the median of the cooking distribution.

Finally, the committee recommends that a sensitivity analysis for the overall risk model be included, in addition to the sensitivity analysis of the individual modules in the exposure continuum.

CONCLUSIONS

The committee does not believe that it is appropriate to offer specific comments regarding the analyses presented in the "Conclusions" section of the Risk Characterization chapter. It believes that it is premature for the draft risk assessment to draw the inferences contained in this section and that its inclusion at this stage of the assessment process conveys an unwarranted confidence in the validity of the model's output. It is more appropriate to include such material after the model has been refined. Alternatively, the level of uncertainty in these conclusions needs to be much more forcefully stated.

The committee believes that recommendations regarding the potential applications of the model's various outputs would be a useful addition to the final risk assessment. The authors should make clear what they believe the model can and cannot be used for. As discussed in Chapter 7 of this review, they should devote particular attention to how anchoring can affect whether particular applications or inferences are appropriate.

GENERAL COMMENTS

The committee notes, as it has elsewhere, that the impact of cross contamination is not assessed in this draft chapter and that characterizations of uncertainty and variability in the results are either weak or absent.

The committee commends the authors for their considerable work in the development of a comprehensive chapter on risk characterization. Although there is much additional work to do to complete the risk characterization, the critical topics have been identified, and initial work presented for each.

REFERENCES

Cassin MH, Lammerding AM, Todd EC, Ross W, McColl RS. 1998. Quantitative risk assessment of *Escherichia coli* O157:H7 in ground beef hamburgers. International Journal of Food Microbiology 41:21–44.

Codex Alimentarius Commission. 1999. Principles and Guidelines for the Conduct of Microbiological Risk Assessment. CAC/GL-30. Food and Agricultural Organization of the United Nations.

FDA/USDA (Food and Drug Administration/US Department of Agriculture). 2001. Draft Assessment of the Relative Risk to Public Health from Foodborne *Listeria monocytogenes* Among Selected Categories of Ready-to-Eat Foods. FDA/Center for Food Safety and Applied Nutrition, USDA/Food Safety and Inspection Service, Centers for Disease Control and Prevention, January 2001. http://www.foodsafety.gov/~dms/lmrisk.html.

ILSI (International Life Sciences Institute). 2000. Revised Framework for Microbial Risk Assessment — An ILSI Risk Science Institute Workshop report. Washington, DC: International Life Sciences Institute.

Marks HM, Coleman ME, Lin CTJ, Roberts T. 1998. Topics in risk assessment: Dynamic flow tree process. Risk Analysis 18:309–328.

WHO (World Health Organization). 1995. Application of Risk Analysis to Food Standards Issues-The report of the Joint FAO/WHO Expert Consultation, 13–17 March 1995 (WHO/FNU/FOS/95.3).

7

Modeling Approach and Implementation

This chapter of the report differs from previous chapters in that it does not directly review a section of the draft *E. coli* O157:H7 risk assessment. Instead, it reviews the basis of the approach and implementation of the model and offers the committee's observations and recommendations regarding it. The discussion thus touches on and overlaps some of the observations offered earlier, as well as providing an overall assessment of the modeling work done to date.

At the outset, it should be said that the effort underlying this risk assessment is impressive. The authors have undertaken an extraordinary task of collection, analysis, and integration of information. It will be an important assessment and will undoubtedly serve as an exemplar for future assessments. The analysts are to be commended for undertaking this work. Nevertheless, several issues remain to be resolved as development continues. The committee notes that the draft's authors have already implemented some of the suggestions discussed below.

The US Department of Agriculture (USDA) Food Safety and Inspection Service (FSIS) effort faced a number of substantial methodologic hurdles whose solutions have not been described in textbooks or in literature peculiar to microbial risk assessment. In addition to methodologic hurdles, the FSIS team has been forced to cope with the inadequacy of the knowledge base. As a result, it is appropriate that they interrupt their risk-assessment effort to allow for peer review and to reassess their solutions to some challenging issues.

The committee commends them both for the magnitude of the effort and for the principles behind their efforts. The committee believes that many of its criticisms and suggestions regarding this model would apply to most previous and current microbial risk-assessment models if they were subject to the same intensity of review.

DESCRIPTION OF THE OVERALL MODELING APPROACH

The approach taken in this modeling effort is to create a highly complex probabilistic simulation model that extends from estimation of the pattern of prevalence of enterohemorrhagic *E. coli* (EHEC) among various types of cattle through propagation of the exposure predictions related to slaughter, processing, and preparation of meals to the estimation of the distribution of dose-response relationships. The dose-response relationships are derived by fitting predicted distributions of exposure to estimates of the population health risk attributable to ground beef as estimated from epidemiologic data.

In its final step, however, the model departs from the standard approach to risk assessment in a way that merits careful attention. Specifically, the risk characterization is carried out in part within the hazard-characterization stage by estimating (on the basis of epidemiologic data and investigations) the annual number of cases of EHEC illness associated with ground beef. Because the dose-response relationship is inferred from an algorithm that was designed to recreate samples from the distribution of the annual number of cases of EHEC illness, the risk estimates provided by the draft model cannot be considered to be independent of the epidemiological data.

Risk Modeling, But Not Risk Assessment as Commonly Understood

A key observation regarding the draft model is that it does not provide a risk assessment in the form that many readers would expect. To label the product a risk assessment implies that the effort is directed toward providing an estimate of risk by collecting evidence and applying mathematical tools; the estimate of risk would be a dependent output of the model. In particular, the use of the terms *farm-to-fork* and *process risk model* will imply to most readers that the many factors involved in the model are aggregated mathematically and propagated forward to generate an estimate of population health risk.

The standard approach to risk assessment is that the information input and the predictive output of the exposure assessment and the dose-response assessment are derived from independent scientific sources and that the dependent output is estimates of risk that are derived from the combination of the two subassessments. With an estimate of risk as the dependent output, the label *risk assessment* is appropriate to describe the analysis in the standard case.

The present modeling effort alters that arrangement by deriving the exposure assessment and the population risk estimates from separate sources and then inferring a dose-response relationship that is mathematically compatible with the calculated exposure assessment and the distribution of population risk estimates. Such a risk assessment might be considered *inverted* because the nominal risk equation *risk = function of (exposure x dose-response relation)* has been reorganized to *dose-response relationship = function of (exposure x risk)*.

An analogy for the present approach may be useful. Consider an analyst estimating the area of a rectangle. The analyst, on the basis of various predictive models, has simulated a distribution of possible lengths of the rectangle. The analyst also has a separate source of information regarding the total area and provides a range of estimates for the area. Given great uncertainty in the width of the rectangle, the analyst decides to generate estimates of the width of the rectangle by dividing samples from the distribution of area by samples from the distribution of length. That generates a set of candidate widths that are compatible with the other two kinds of information. In an analogous way, the *area* assessment is inverted to become a *width* assessment. Moving forward, the analyst uses the estimates of length and the derived set of widths to generate estimates of area. The questions faced in this situation are whether the calculation in the model should be described as providing an estimate of area, whether and how the model can be validated, and what can be inferred (statistically) from the set of width estimates generated in the process and how they can be used. If we modify the length or width of the rectangle in some way by using a management strategy, is it reasonable to estimate the resulting area simply by multiplying the new length by the inferred widths?

For the FSIS assessment, the question is whether and how the inferred dose-response relationship can be used in future assessments and management planning to predict the benefits (in terms of risk reduction) of altering ground-beef production, delivery, or preparation.

Assessment of the Rationale for the Inverted Assessment Approach

The nonstandard treatment of dose-response assessment appears to be based on the judgment that this component of the risk estimation carries the most—and least likely to be resolved—uncertainty. Furthermore, the uncertainty in the dose-response relationship is judged to be less than the uncertainty in the population risk estimate that typically would be considered the goal of the risk-assessment effort. That judgment seems reasonable in light of practical and ethical constraints in performing human dose-response experiments and the continued lack of high-quality evidence suitable for dose-response characterization from, for example, outbreak investigations.

The departure from the standard approach can be justified, in principle, by the assertion that the primary goal of risk assessment is better understanding of the mechanisms of the generation, transmission, and attenuation of risk through the system. To be considered appropriate, that goal would have to be considered more important than providing an estimate of population health risk that is derived solely from simulation of the components of the risk-generating system.

Once it has established and communicated an appropriately limited set of goals (and acknowledged that not all the candidate goals can be equally served by the same effort), the decisions made by the modeling group to use various techniques can be understood and judged relative to the stated goals rather than to a presumed or standard goal.

In light of the concerns raised in the earlier sections of this review, particularly those addressing the Production and Slaughter Modules, the authors may wish to reconsider whether the dose-response assessment is truly the most uncertain modular component of the model. From a modeling perspective, the current state of knowledge available to predict the transmission and ultimate fate of EHEC from the farm to the ground-beef patty may be at least as uncertain as the dose-response relationship. Given the complexity of the steps involved, combined with the legal and regulatory data-collection and -reporting environment, there may be little hope of gaining insight into this process without a fundamental change in the situation.

It may be possible to place more faith in the use of *Shigella dysenteriae* 1 as a surrogate for the best estimate of a dose-response function for EHEC, as is proposed in the Hazard Characterization chapter, than in the implemented exposure model as a surrogate for the reality of the ecology and transmission of EHEC within and between farms, feedlots, slaughterhouses, combo bins, and grinders and through the multitude of potential cooking practices and consumer behaviors.

An Example of the Standard Approach

After the FSIS draft report was released for public comment, a risk assessment by Nauta and colleagues (2001) became available. It addresses the risk of EHEC illness from steak tartare consumption in the Netherlands and was produced for the Rijksinstituut voor Volksgezondheid en Milieu (RIVM). The risk assessment had not been peer-reviewed when it became available to the committee, but it is described in sufficient detail to compare the modeling efforts at the level of the overall approach. Nauta et al. carry out the risk assessment in the more standard format, providing independent estimates of the distribution of exposure through predictive modeling and of the dose-response relationship on the basis of data from a 1997 outbreak in Japan (Shinagawa, 1997). Those are combined to form a prediction of the population health risk attributable to consumption of steak tartare contaminated with EHEC. The results of the analysis can be compared on a truly independent basis with population risk estimates from the Netherlands. In this case, the baseline predicted number of cases of EHEC illness due to steak tartare is higher than the total number of cases associated with EHEC from all foods. That independent assessment demonstrates that some components of the model are overstating the risk. The point of this comparison is to suggest that there may be some merits of "face-value" validation in which the model generates a risk estimate independent of illness surveillance data. The Nauta et al. model may not be satisfactory in its performance, but it has the considerable potential benefit of independent and transparent validation.

The FSIS risk model cannot provide that degree of output validation until the dose-response relationship is generated from a source independent of the validation data. It would also be possible to validate the model if one or more surrogate dose-response relationships (for a foodborne pathogen other than O157:H7) were adopted for use. Alternatively, it is possible to validate the inferred dose-response function as was attempted in the Risk Characterization chapter with an outbreak investigation. Regardless of any validation efforts, transparency would be greatly improved by a simple demonstration of the range of risk estimates that are generated by using a variety of dose-response relationships (such as the upper and lower bounds of the dose-response envelope) to show the performance and the sensitivity of the model in various possible dose-response scenarios.

The committee notes that the RIVM model is not included here as an example of a better model. Its authors acknowledge many limitations, and the analysis is of a much smaller scope and less detail with respect to the evidence base. However, it is included as an example of a model that provides a risk estimate as a dependent outcome and that would more closely match the standard definition of *risk assessment*. Having maintained separation between the risk assessment and the national surveillance data, the RIVM model has the benefit that its output can be compared with independent epidemiologic data for purposes of validation.

Additional Comments Regarding the Inverted Approach

The alternative approach used by FSIS carries some disadvantages. As noted, the primary drawback is the loss of the face-value validation of the output through comparison with independent epidemiologic data, in that the data have essentially become part of the assessment. The impact of the inverted assessment is that—from the point of view of comparison with population health risk data—the model can never be wrong (because it constitutes a circular argument). An overestimate in the exposure distribution would be accommodated by underestimating the probability of illness, and underestimation in the exposure distribution could be accommodated by overestimating the probability of illness. The committee assumes that the motivation behind the algorithm is to practice a form of model updating, that is, using independent observation to improve the accuracy of the model. The updating algorithms are described later, including some suggestions for making the updating more compatible with these goals.

Another drawback in the approach is the lack of a scientific evidence base for the dose-response relationship. The dose-response relationship is derived from model assumptions that are not related to the pathogenicity of EHEC. Any change in the parameters of the exposure assessment (for example, an improved estimate of the prevalence in a population of cattle) or in the assumptions leading to the baseline population health risk estimate (for example, a change in the etiologic fraction estimates) changes the basis of the inferred dose-response relationship. It is not clear where an appropriate end to this cycle of revision would be.

The approach is much harder to understand than a straightforward assessment. The resulting uncertainty in the simulated dose-response parameters is a product of the uncertainty in the exposure assessment and the uncertainty in the population health risk estimate. The only information provided in the algorithm that is directly related to the issue of the pathogenicity of EHEC is the envelope that limits the search space in inferring the dose-response function and the assumption that the functional form will be beta-Poisson. The complexity of the relationship between the many sources of uncertainty and the final distribution of dose-response parameters may be a threat to *real* transparency for the great majority of external reviewers. This is a different matter from the *strict* transparency of the approach demonstrated through provision of the report, appendixes, and underlying model code. Some judgment is required as to whether a dose-response relationship derived in this way is preferable to a simpler model with a more transparent depiction of the underlying uncertainty.

Despite the potential problems, it must be recognized that the mere departure from a standard approach does not in itself constitute an error. A decision to depart from the standard approach could be considered entirely appropriate to the situation. But, it is important to communicate the nature of the departure and its impact on the overall utility of the model and to ensure that readers do not misunderstand the output of the model as being a risk assessment as it is commonly understood.

Regardless of the presence of any technical errors, there is the risk of errors of omission and commission. The potential error of omission lies in failing to ensure the full communication of these issues. The potential error of commission lies in describing the effort as "generating" or "predicting" population risk estimates when in fact population risk estimates are provided as input to the model on the basis of epidemiologic data.

A serious miscommunication could result if readers form the impression that the model propagates evidence forward to generate population health risks and then judge the model to be appropriate on the basis of the quality of the match to what are thought to be independent epidemiologic data. Having departed from the standard approach, the authors have the burden of ensuring that readers do not construct an inappropriate mental model of the approach and thereby form a judgment of its validity.

There may also be some concern about the utility of a model generated in this way if risk-management decision-making requires the provision of a risk-assessment model that can be validated to some extent by national-level epidemiologic data. Such a requirement is not stated for this situation.

Therefore the committee recommends that the authors communicate more clearly the nature of, the rationale for, and the impact of the departure from the standard risk-assessment approach and should consider relabeling the product as a *system risk model* to avoid implying that the model generates an estimate of risk independent of that derived from epidemiologic data.

The authors should reconsider the approach taken to infer the dose-response relationship in light of the loss of the potential for model-output validation, a desire to improve transparency, and concerns regarding whether the uncertainty is actually greatest in the dose-response characterization. Chapter 5 of this report offers comments regarding the choice of surrogate pathogens.

DESCRIPTION OF
MODEL-UPDATING (ANCHORING) ALGORITHMS

At several points in the development of the model, algorithms are invoked to adjust the simulation outputs of the model to make them more compatible with observed data. This approach, called "anchoring" in the draft, is applied at the end of the simulation of grinder loads to adjust the simulation results to be compatible with FSIS sampling data. A variation of model updating is also applied in the hazard characterization stage to match simulated exposure distributions with predictions of the numbers of cases of illness.

The application of model updating is well founded in health risk assessment and related fields of environmental modeling (see Brand and Small, 1995; Small and Fischbeck, 1999). Updating is of particular value when models are created under conditions of high levels of uncertainty. In such cases, the variance in model estimates grows as the evidence is propagated through each linked submodel. In the end, the distribution representing uncertainty in the predicted risk can be too broad to provide discriminating evidence in support of decisions. Thus, it is generally desirable to include any source of information that can reduce uncertainty in a model's output. The algorithms for model updating used in the draft report are described below.

Updating Grinder-Load Concentrations

The exposure-assessment modules yield distributions for the number of grinder loads predicted to contain levels of EHEC ranging from 1 colony-forming unit (CFU) to 10^{12} CFU. FSIS carries out microbiologic testing for *E. coli* O157:H7 in raw ground beef, so there is an opportunity to provide additional information to the model by using the results of the sampling.

The approach taken is as follows:

1. Infer the distribution of the proportion of positive samples taken from grinders that would be statistically consistent with the FSIS sampling evidence.

2. Calculate (by simulation) the proportion of positive samples by simulating the exposure model up to the point of grinder-load concentration and simulating the sampling and detection process.

3. For each simulation, compare the calculated proportion of positive samples with the distribution of the proportion of positive samples inferred from FSIS results.

Each simulation is treated in one of three ways:

- If the simulated prevalence falls between the 5th and 95th percentile of the inferred prevalence distribution, it is accepted as a plausible simulation.
- If the simulated prevalence exceeds the 95th percentile of the inferred prevalence distribution, the simulation is rejected from future calculations as implausible.
- If the simulated prevalence is below the 5th percentile of the in-

ferred prevalence distribution, the simulation is amended by shifting the histogram of grinder-load concentrations to the right (that is, increasing it in 0.5 log increments) until the calculated proportion of positive samples approximates the mean of the inferred proportion of positive samples.

That approach raises a number of concerns in that it contains arbitrary measures and unsupported suppositions:

- The choice of the 5th and 95th percentiles of the distribution as critical limits is arbitrary and effectively censors or distorts data that fall outside these bounds.
- The uncertainty in the range of proportions inferred from the sampling evidence may be underestimated. Specifically, the inference uses a point estimate of the sensitivity of the detection set at exactly 4 times the point estimate of the sensitivity of another test that is itself uncertain. The effect is to overestimate the inferential value of the FSIS sampling process and therefore to limit artificially the acceptable range of exposure simulations.
- The distinction made to accept and adjust simulations below 5% and to reject unconditionally those above 95% appears arbitrary. One could just as easily find a mechanistic justification to adjust the concentration histogram downward as to adjust it upward.
- The fabrication process is modeled as contributing to grinder loads only in situations in which other uncertain factors may be underestimating the pathogen load in grinders, as opposed to having an independent contribution in each simulation, as might be expected; in this way, the impact of fabrication depends on unrelated factors and not on any explicit assumptions regarding the process of fabrication.
- The shift of all grinder-load profiles that fall below the 5th percentile toward a distribution leading to the mean proportion is an arbitrary distortion of the grinder concentration distribution.
- The overall effect of the algorithm is to limit the simulations to those which are compatible with the central portion of the sampling evidence and to distort other simulations to reinforce the mean estimate from the sampling evidence. This is particularly problematic in that it eliminates lower-probability high-risk situations, which are normally of great interest in risk assessment.
- Generally speaking, the parameters of the dose-response algorithm are not well specified, making it difficult to understand and evaluate the derivation.

The draft does not provide summary statistics associated with the proportion of simulations that are accepted, rejected, or adjusted. It is therefore not possible to judge how large an impact the algorithm has on the overall simulation process. In addition, there does not appear to be an analysis of the factors underlying the rejection of simulations—that is, an assessment of the patterns of inputs that are associated with the set of rejected or adjusted simulations. The draft's Appendix A refers to a paper on a Bayesian synthesis method by Green et al. (2000) as a source for the procedure, but the inferential approach described in the paper does not appear to have been used.

Estimating the Dose-Response Relationship

The process for estimating the dose-response relationship is based on iterative matching of two pieces of evidence. In each iteration, the first source of evidence is a sample from a set of simulated exposure distributions. Each simulation generates a histogram of the frequency of servings at discrete levels of number of CFU per serving. The second source of evidence is 19 percentile estimates (from 5% to 95%, in 5% increments) from an uncertainty distribution of the population risk estimate of the annual number of illnesses, on the basis of epidemiologic analysis. The assumed dose-response curve is the beta-Poisson function with parameters α and ID_{50}.

A fitting algorithm then finds a value for ID_{50} that will translate each exposure distribution into each of the 19 discrete estimates of population risk. This process is repeated for seven potential values of the α parameter. The result is a total of $19 \times 7 \times N$ dose-response relationships (combinations of α and ID_{50}) where N is the number of simulated exposure distributions for which the fitting is done (N appears to be set at 100).

The percentiles of the ID_{50} parameter are then calculated from the entire pool of results. This is not specified in the report, but the median dose-response curve appears to be based on the 50th percentile from the pool of ID_{50} values. The value of α that is assumed to apply for the "50th percentile" dose-response curve is not clear after a review of both the model implementation and the draft.

The committee has the following concerns with this approach:

- There is no description of the mathematical or statistical basis of the approach, nor is there any reference to a similar approach applied elsewhere in the literature.
- The basis of including the 19 percentiles for developing a pool of ID_{50} values is not clear; it appears to be arbitrary.
- The meaning of an ID_{50} value that is the 50th percentile of such a pool of fitting results is not clear and is not explained beyond the state-

ment that it is the median value of a pool of data whose elements do not appear to have a formal basis.
- The approach does not appear to conform to any established process of inference. Some reference is made in the spreadsheet to prior and posterior estimates, implying a Bayesian updating process, but no evidence of a likelihood function or other expected components of such an inferential approach is given.
- Although it may be reasonable on scientific and qualitative grounds to state that a pair of surrogate pathogens form a plausible envelope, this is not equivalent to stating that the values of α and ID_{50} must be limited to those achieved by the fitting algorithm for the two pathogens. The uncertainty in the values of both α and ID_{50} that result from fitting to the feeding-trial data for *Shigella* and enteropathogenic *E. coli* would be expected to be broad. In the dose-response estimation method, the range of uncertainty in the α parameter is limited to 0.16–0.22 in steps of 0.01, thereby providing seven alternative values of α. That is particularly relevant, given the committee's finding that *Shigella dysenteriae* 1 may constitute a reasonable surrogate for a "best estimate," rather than its current role as an estimate of the upper bound of the envelope.

Alternative Model-Updating Strategies

Both the model-updating processes described above appear to lack a formal statistical basis. Given the use of Bayesian updating processes at various points in the model and the overall reliance on Monte Carlo simulation, it seems appropriate to consider using a form of Bayesian Monte Carlo simulation (or some of its more advanced resampling relatives) to incorporate properly the information provided by the observational data (see, for example, Brand and Small, 1995; Dilks et al., 1992; Gelman et al., 1995; Small and Fischbeck, 1999).

There are a number of key differences in the application of an algorithm based on the Bayesian Monte Carlo methods:

- It does not place the burden of model adjustment on any one part of the model (that is, both the exposure and dose-response modules would be updated).
- The updating process works both "upstream" and "downstream" of the observation point.
- It does not allow for arbitrary adjustments.
- The quality of the process generating the observational data must be carefully scrutinized and quantified in the development of likelihood functions.

- It can be appended to the simulation model with moderate computational effort.
- The sensitivity of the results to the updating process can be studied and compared with intuitive judgment regarding the true informativeness of the observational data.
- It allows the simulation model to deviate from the distribution of observations of the output to the extent that the observations of the output are themselves imperfect.
- Prior statements of uncertainty (such as the dose-response envelope) are provided for but with more formal treatment.

Therefore the committee recommends that the authors replace the current algorithms for updating grinder-load concentrations with a more formal, statistically based model updating procedure.

Also, the committee recommends that the authors replace the current algorithms for calculating dose-response parameters with model elements based on evidence that is independent of national epidemiologic data. That will allow for limited validation of model estimates with epidemiologic data. For the grinder-level observational data and any other observational data in the system being simulated, the authors may wish to consider Bayesian Monte Carlo methods to provide a structured method of updating model parameters in light of observational data.

MODEL VALIDATION

At several points, the FSIS draft report argues that its findings are "comparable" with other estimates or descriptions of outbreaks. In some cases, however, the comparisons are unconvincing. The draft cites Cassin and colleagues' (1998) mean per-serving risk of 5.1×10^{-5} as being "comparable" with the report's finding of 9.6×10^{-7}. Using the same calculation that converts 18.2 billion servings into 17,500 cases of illness in the draft risk assessment, the Cassin et al. result would yield 930,000 cases. That is clearly not "comparable." It is thus unclear what the criteria might be for assigning such a label. If the results are comparable in some other ways, they should be described, but the purely numerical results suggest just the opposite.

Apart from numerically questionable comparisons, the underlying basis of comparison is also problematic and has substantial potential for miscommunication. The draft model is constrained to deliver risk estimates that are predicted by epidemiologic analysis. The comparison may also suggest that the underlying models are comparable. In reality, the comparison is between the Cassin model and the epidemiologic analysis. On that basis, the Cassin model substantially overestimates the risk com-

MODELING APPROACH AND IMPLEMENTATION 109

pared with that suggested by the epidemiologic analysis. At the same time, little can be said in comparing the Cassin model with the underlying draft model, because of the inverted assessment approach.

It is stated that the derived dose-response function "shows consistency with information obtained in a ground-beef associated outbreak in the northwestern United States" (p. 119 in the draft). On the basis of the draft's Figure 4-5, the information obtained from the ground-beef-associated outbreak is so dispersed that it is consistent with virtually every dose-response curve that could reasonably be suggested. It appears that the outbreak provides hardly any discriminatory information with respect to choosing or validating a range of dose-response curves. Use of the label "consistency" may be somewhat generous with respect to the implied validation. If anything, the information from the outbreak suggests that the dose-response envelope is too limiting, as acknowledged by the statement (p. 119 in the draft) that the "*Shigella dysenteriae* dose-response function fails to explain all of the outbreak's uncertainty."

The committee recommends that the authors reconsider the basis of model validation and avoid implying a greater degree of validation than is warranted by the comparisons presented.

MODELING ISSUES IN HAZARD CHARACTERIZATION

One of the goals of the risk assessment is to provide a measure of the opportunity to reduce risk through various risk mitigation actions. Assumptions used in a hazard characterization can have a great impact on the ability of a model to represent the expected value of mitigations accurately.

Scope and Context Decisions in Hazard Characterization

A number of important subassessments are required in hazard identification and hazard characterization:

- *To describe the evidence for probability of illness as a function of any risk factors (that is, dose, age, disease states or other conditions of the host, sex, and food-matrix effects).* In the draft risk assessment, the probability of illness is provided as a function of dose, but no other variables are used to modify the probability. Admittedly, the evidence base to support modification of the probability of illness as a function of factors other than dose is weak. However, other risk factors might be included if the hazard characterization were simplified—specifically, if it were based on the probability of illness given an exposure event as opposed to exposure to a particular dose. That could provide improved resolution in one part of the analysis—the ability to explain demographic differences in the probability of illness. However, it would come at the cost of losing the benefits associated with explicit dose dependence in the probability of illness.

- *To describe the full spectrum of more-severe health outcomes that can result from the primary illness and their relationship with any risk factors (dose, age, pre-existing disease states, sex, and the like).* The draft risk assessment does not use any risk factors in calculating the likelihood of transition from illness to more-severe outcomes, such as hemolytic uremic syndrome (HUS) or death, although evidence of these variations is cited. The number of severe outcomes is taken to be a fraction of the total number of cases, with no specific allocation of the burden of the severe outcomes to particular exposure groups, such as children or the elderly. The implications of the simplification are discussed in more detail below.

- *To describe the likelihood of secondary infections as a function of the same risk factors (dose, age, disease state, sex, and so on), including the potential for secondary infection without primary illness.* Without calculating the risk of secondary infection (presumably by incorporating particular risk factors for secondary infection, such as age), it is not possible to represent accurately the public-health benefit associated with avoiding the primary cases. For example, the draft suggests that the etiologic fraction associated with ground beef may be lower for children because they are also exposed to secondary infections from day-care facilities. The latter is true, but it does not necessary imply that reductions aimed at children will reduce a smaller proportion of the problem. Given that the initial EHEC exposure in the day-care environment is likely to be traceable ultimately to some animal reservoir (such as farm exposure, pets, and waterborne and foodborne vehicles), each primary case prevented among children could have substantially more benefit in terms of the number and severity of secondary cases than in terms of prevention of a primary case among adults.

- *To provide an indication of the relative value to be placed on preventing primary cases that are more likely to result in severe morbidity or death or on preventing cases in subpopulations that are generally afforded more protection in public-health efforts (for example, children).* Evaluation of the relative value of interventions is particularly important where there is known heterogeneity of the case-complication or case-fatality rates across subpopulations. That is true for the *E. coli* O157:H7 infection case-complication rates for HUS and the case-fatality rates with and without HUS in the very young and the very old. Because the *increased likelihood of secondary infection* among the very young is coupled with the *increased likelihood of developing HUS*, these factors combine to make up an important potential source of health burden that is missing from the draft model.

The committee believes that there are a number of reasons why it would be valuable to provide a detailed characterization of the risk attributable to ground beef or to beef and dairy production generally. To characterize fully the risk assessment and its relationship to public-health goals, the following are required:

• An explicit accounting of the total risk attributable to the pathogen regardless of source.

• An explicit accounting of the proportion (and uncertainty therein) of the risk that is available to be reduced through mitigation of sources and pathways that are included in the risk assessment. This characterization is valuable in any risk assessment, but it is vital in this case, where the estimate of risk attributable to ground-beef consumption is integrated directly into the model to derive estimates of the dose-response function.

• An explicit accounting of the proportion of risk (admittedly, very uncertain) that is thought to be attributable to pathways that are not part of the scope of this assessment but are closely related (EHEC other than O157:H7, cross contamination in homes and in food services, unpasteurized milk, occupational exposure, waterborne risk due to livestock operations, contact with animals, custom slaughter, manure management, and so on). This would allow for the consideration of the appropriateness of the scope of the assessment with particular attention to missing pathways that generate health benefits from the same mitigation options as are being considered for the pathways that are included in the scope (for example, reduction of the pathogen prevalence or load in animal reservoirs).

• An explicit accounting of the proportion of secondary cases (for example, among children) that might be prevented by avoidance of primary cases (caused by consumption of contaminated ground beef) that are within the scope of the risk assessment.

• An explicit accounting of the various indicators of attributable risk (outbreak data, case-control studies of sporadic cases, passive surveillance, and the like) and their expected inferential value as related to a particular food and pathogen combination.

• An explicit accounting of the potential for increased variability in the attributable risk with season and region. For example, an increase in human cases in summer could be a result of more contact through swimming, increased pathogen loads in drinking-water supplies because of rainfall or snowmelt patterns, increased contact with animals and surface water, and more contact with untreated drinking water at cottages and camps. Those factors are outside the risk assessment, but they may influence the observed patterns of incidence of *E. coli* O157:H7 illness and could provide important context for the management of the problem.

• An explicit accounting of the potential for different patterns of attributable risk of illnesses (in particular, those in sensitive subpopulations) that are more likely to have severe sequelae.

Such information will be highly uncertain, but its absence seriously undermines the ability to assess and characterize risks and to measure the full value of potential mitigations. It is thus a major component of the contextual description of the risk assessment that would be key to the understanding of the situation by risk managers and stakeholders.

The following hypothetical example illustrates the point (the numbers are chosen for illustrative purposes only):

Product X accounts for 20% (20,000) of all EHEC illness. These illnesses have a case-complication rate of 5%, resulting in 1,000 cases of HUS.

Now consider two scenarios with respect to risk attribution—A1 and A2.

> A1: Product X accounts for 20% (20,000 cases) of illness, and the attribution is constant among different age groups.
> A2: Product X accounts for 40% of EHEC illnesses in children but only 10% in the remainder of the population.

And consider two scenarios with respect to attribution of the disease burden—C1 and C2.

> C1: The case rate and the case-HUS rate are uniform in the population.
> C2: Of the 20,000 cases, 8,000 occur in children, and the case-HUS rate for children is 10% (800 cases of HUS). The other 12,000 illnesses occur in the general population with a case-HUS rate of 1.67% (200 cases).

And consider two scenarios with respect to the utility of preventing complicated versus uncomplicated cases—U1 and U2.

> U1: Equal weight is placed on preventing cases, whether they are likely to result in severe outcomes or not.
> U2: Preventing of cases leading to HUS is considered to be 1,000 times more valuable to society than preventing uncomplicated cases (self-limiting gastroenteritis).

Different combinations of those scenarios produce different risk-management situations and involve various levels of focus on particular population groups. If the burden of HUS and other serious complications is a large part of the basis of risk-management decision-making, it is important that the risk assessment explicitly incorporate scenarios that address them. That can be achieved by demonstrating which of a set of composite scenarios best represents reality or by allowing for multiple scenarios and addressing the alternative assumptions in the risk characterization and the risk assessment in general.

If all those issues are explicit, it becomes much clearer how the draft risk assessment and hypothetical mitigations will affect public health. This includes the gains achieved by reducing the prevalence of contaminated product entering the home or retail preparation environment and thereby reducing exposure via cross contamination. It also includes the gains associated with prevention of secondary transmission by elimination of primary cases that have foodborne sources. In addition, the predicted health benefits can be added to or compared with benefits associated with EHEC control in animal reservoirs apart from the impact on the food supply (including animal contact, waterborne transmission, occupational exposure, and secondary cases that stem from these primary sources). It would be unfortunate if the full value of the potential effectiveness of proposed mitigations were underestimated because of limitations in the scope of the assessment.

Therefore the committee recommends that the authors review the scope and allocation of effort in the risk-assessment model with respect to its ability to generate unique insight into the burden of hemolytic uremic syndrome, other severe sequelae, and mortality. Those are the outcomes that arguably justify the attention paid to EHEC compared with pathogens that result in a much larger number of illnesses. The authors should also review the scope of the model and its documentation to ensure that the full public-health context and thereby the value of potential mitigations can be described and measured by the risk assessment.

Attribution of EHEC to Ground-Beef Consumption

The FSIS draft risk assessment relies on matching the cases predicted by the broad spectrum of ground-beef production and consumption behaviors (although ignoring, at this point in development, the potential for cross contamination) with the fraction of cases that might be prevented by removal of the risk factor of eating "pink" ground beef. Given that the epidemiologic data effectively become part of the dose-response assessment and ultimately govern the risk estimates, they need to be afforded detailed treatment.

The fraction attributable to ground beef is calculated on the basis of three sources of information:

- The proportion of outbreaks attributable to ground beef (one calculation).

- The proportion of illnesses within these outbreaks that are associated with ground beef (one calculation).
- The population-attributable risk calculated from case-control studies of sporadic cases (four calculations).

Those six calculations are used in the model to estimate the proportion of cases attributable to ground beef by randomly selecting draws in each iteration, assuming that the true fraction is equally likely to be one of the six calculated estimates.

There are a number of concerns with respect to each of the sources of information and their use in the draft risk assessment:

- The information on the proportion of outbreaks attributable to ground beef and the proportion of outbreak cases should be applied only to the fraction of EHEC cases that are believed to occur in the form of outbreaks. This also applies to information based on sporadic cases.
- Outbreaks whose source is not identified are allocated equally among known sources. Consideration should be given to the notion that outbreaks with unknown sources are far less likely to originate in ground beef, given that ground beef is a leading candidate in any investigation of EHEC outbreaks.
- For the case-control studies, the logic applied is that only cases that resulted from exposures of persons who recall consuming "pink-in-the-middle" ground beef are attributable to ground beef; other cases are not. That does not take into account the probability of illness associated with any other consumption of undercooked ground beef, including respondents that did not notice the color of the meat and circumstances in which the meat was not pink but had surviving organisms.
- An unpublished paper by Kassenborg et al. (2001) cited in the draft gives the population attributable risk (PAR) as 8% and 7%, respectively, for the risk factors "ate pink hamburger at home" and "ate pink hamburger away from home." Because removal of both pathways of exposure would reduce the number of cases associated with ground-beef consumption, it would seem that they should be added in the calculation of the fraction associated with ground beef. These fractions are averaged in the draft analysis, yielding a lower limit of 7.5% for the PAR instead of their sum of 15%. It seems reasonable that the risk attributable to exposures to beef known to be "pink in the middle" should constitute a minimum for the attribution of total risk to ground-beef consumption. Such exposure seems to account for only a subset of the exposures to contaminated ground beef even if the estimation is limited to direct consumption of ground meat as opposed to consumption involving cross contamination.

- The risk factor "pink ground beef" could be confounded (as suggested in the Kassenborg et al. manuscript) with cross contamination if there is a common causal source, such as poorly trained food preparers or inattention to food-safety practices.

During one of the committee's public meetings, comments were received regarding the use of Centers for Disease Control and Prevention (CDC) outbreak data in the estimation of the fraction of EHEC that is attributable to ground beef. [The comments were in the form of a letter and a copy of DeWaal et al. (2001) provided by the Center for Science in the Public Interest.] The comments included the suggestion that the draft report underestimates the attributable risk by estimating the proportion of outbreaks and cases as a fraction of all outbreaks (including, for example, those with waterborne sources). The committee notes that the choice of outbreaks and cases from *all sources* is the appropriate denominator because FSIS is using this estimate to infer an attributable number of cases from the FoodNet surveillance system, which itself includes illnesses from *all sources*. Use of *foodborne sources* to generate a proportional estimate and *all sources* from FoodNet would lead to overestimation of the number of cases attributable to ground beef, assuming that all other factors were unbiased. Nonetheless, estimates of the attributable fractions of foodborne outbreaks and foodborne cases would provide valuable context.

Comments were also received regarding the completeness of the CDC outbreak database. Some consideration should be given to the likelihood and magnitude of any bias that may result in attributable risk estimates from exclusion of outbreaks that are not contained in CDC databases. Again, clarification of the estimated proportion of EHEC illnesses that appear to be in the form of detectable outbreaks would put this issue into better perspective.

Therefore the committee recommends that the USDA or perhaps an interagency body consider developing a standard and formal procedure for estimating the fractions of foodborne illnesses attributable to different foods. This will need to take into account the diverse and often conflicting sources of evidence available, including expert judgment. The process should be carried out independently from the process of commodity-pathogen-specific risk assessment and should be continuously updated.

SOFTWARE IMPLEMENTATION

The FSIS draft risk model consists of the evidence base captured in the documentation and a simulation model implemented with the spreadsheet environment Microsoft Excel (referred to hereafter as Excel). The simulation model is implemented by using Monte Carlo simulation. The model was provided to the committee in multiple versions:

- A version that uses probabilistic sampling functions that are part of an Excel add-in, @RISK, with the overall simulation process controlled by macros written with Visual Basic for Applications (VBA).
- A version that uses probabilistic sampling functions provided by FSIS, with both the sampling functions and the overall simulation model implemented with VBA (no longer requiring @RISK).

Choice of Modeling Environment

In the field of quantitative risk assessment, and for quantitative microbial risk assessment in particular, the use of Excel as a modeling environment is very common. The @RISK add-in is also a common tool for probabilistic simulation in quantitative risk assessment. These choices for software implementation are associated with various benefits, costs, and risks.

Benefits:
The basic modeling environment (Excel) is one of the most widely used software programs in the world. That makes sharing of the basic model structure accessible to a great majority of interested parties with no incremental cost for the broader community. To the extent that there is value in having model assumptions and calculations visible to the largest possible audience, Excel serves this purpose. However, as discussed below, Excel without the benefit of modeling "add-ins" does not provide the capacity to perform probabilistic simulation. And, the spreadsheet environment is inherently problematic for the purposes of complex modeling.

For simulation models of low to moderate complexity, a majority of interested parties and potential reviewers can follow the flow of information and calculation in a spreadsheet. It is reasonable to assume that stakeholders who cannot readily follow spreadsheet logic have ready access to someone who can assist them. In this case, there is great value to the broader community in having an implementation that does not present barriers to transparency.

Another benefit of using commonly available software is that the quality of the software is to some extent known. The quality may be criticized in some cases (for example, because of problems with random-number generation algorithms or inaccuracies that are known to occur in specific situations), but the large community of users of such software essentially acts as informal quality assurance. It may be tempting to replace widely used software with software that is superior in some particular function, but that could come at the cost of a lower (or effectively unknown) level of quality assurance in other functions. There is essentially a risk–risk tradeoff in the choice of software.

Costs:

Excel does not provide algorithms to invoke and control a sample-and-calculate iteration process (to automatically repeat calculations with new random samples) and to store and process the simulation results (such as displaying and providing the average value obtained in a set of 10,000 sample-and-calculate iterations). The sampling and simulation control functionality is provided by various software packages as add-ins to Excel (such as @RISK and Crystal Ball). The add-ins generally cost more than $500 and present a financial barrier to widespread dissemination and review of the models among stakeholders. For stakeholders who have an interest in exploring the model but do not have a long-term interest in quantitative risk assessment with spreadsheets, that constitutes a substantial one-time cost to review and run the model. Software packages that allow for models to be viewed and simulated by others at no cost would be beneficial in addressing the problem.

For probabilistic modeling, good practice (Burmaster and Anderson, 1994) suggests the use of so-called second-order modeling that explicitly separates uncertainty (representing a deficiency in the knowledge base) and variability (representing known dispersion or distribution of some quantity). That requires an additional level of complexity in the control of the calculations (loops within loops) that is not available in the standard recalculation of spreadsheets and is only crudely available in @RISK. To implement that functionality in Excel, the USDA team has written VBA code to control the ordering of the calculations and the storage of the considerable amount of data generated (and for other reasons). Including VBA code in the overall simulation reduces the overall transparency of the model in proportion to the ability of reviewers to understand the workings of this programming language and the amount of time they have available for such review.

Risks:

The basic spreadsheet environment has several limitations. As models become more and more complex, the amount of spreadsheet space taken up by the model assumptions needed for intermediate calculations and the storage of output calculations becomes quite large. That can be managed with VBA code to store and perform intermediate calculations, careful documentation of the spreadsheet, and detailed user manuals. However, beyond some level of complexity, the spreadsheet environment becomes more a problem than a solution for the purposes of model communication. The benefits of using widely available spreadsheet software, noted above, can be outweighed by the inadequacy of spreadsheets in the management and communication of complex models.

The popularity of spreadsheets is based largely on the user's freedom to structure and implement calculations in diverse ways with little or no formal structure. In addition, it is possible to directly access and control the data and the calculations with relative ease. Such freedom brings considerable systematic risk. The risk is based on the accessibility of individual data points (in large arrays and matrices) and the potential for undetected data corruption or formula errors that may be singular faults in a large array of otherwise correct formulas. It is a considerable challenge to ensure that the data and formulas are uncorrupted by small errors, particularly when multiple persons are implementing and adjusting the model.

The basic problem with spreadsheets is that they make it easy for an analyst to make errors. Spreadsheets lack the transparency of explicit programs. Simply put, it can be hard to keep track of what values depend on what other values and to trace an error in a spreadsheet because the structure of the calculations is cryptic. The interconnections between subcomponents of the model (workbooks) can be difficult to follow because all variables are global variables. Software developed in a modern computer language explicitly lists the input and output variables used by a particular model component. If one component's variables are to be used by another component, this is usually handled through an explicit list of formal parameters. It is also hard to document updates or changes of a spreadsheet; this makes spreadsheets especially cumbersome when multiple analysts participate in developing the calculations.

In some cases, there can be no assurance other than through exhaustive checking of all individual cells and formulas. This process can be time-consuming and generally requires expert knowledge of the model's intentions. The audit process is itself error-prone because of the combination of the complexity and monotony of the exercise. The task is made more difficult in the draft model by the use of direct cell references as opposed to the use of named identifiers to refer to another quantity in the model; for example, a formula for microbial growth uses the spreadsheet cell location *Temperatures!$AB$82*, which is located on another worksheet, instead of the label "CookingTemperature" to refer to the cooking temperature. The draft authors indicate (in Appendix C) that direct cell referencing was used to ease the audit process, but it is difficult to understand how it makes the task easier. The situation is complicated if one tries to explore the Visual Basic code, in which a different reference system ("cell(*row*, *column*)") is used. The extreme cumbersomeness and error-prone nature of these multiple ways of referring to a variable are perhaps sufficient in themselves to justify the effort to rework the simulation model in an alternative environment.

The committee and an external reviewer had considerable difficulty in following the information flow in the model. Several errors in the spreadsheets are noted in an independent review prepared by Edmund Crouch, which appears as Appendix D of this report.

Choice of Sampling Engine (@RISK versus VBA)

As stated above, two versions of the draft model were provided to the committee. The versions differ in the software that converts input assumptions for the distribution of inputs into random samples that are used to construct the output distributions. The choice to use custom VBA code to generate random numbers provides the benefit of independence from @RISK and generates risks generally associated with new or unproven code.

Benefits of independence from @RISK:
- A much larger community of potential model collaborators and reviewers.
- Avoidance of the costs associated with @RISK (for USDA and people interested in using, collaborating on, or reviewing the model).
- A higher level of transparency because the sampling and simulation code for @RISK is proprietary and therefore cannot be openly scrutinized.

Risks in new and unproven simulation code:
- Costs associated with continued development and quality assurance of the simulation code.
- Version control (ensuring that all copies of the spreadsheet have the same error-free simulation code).
- A lower level of "informal" quality control, given the much-reduced numbers of users and reviewers.
- The limited value of transparency in the simulation code if it is not expertly scrutinized and compared with alternatives.
- The loss of various additional current and future features of tools like @RISK (graphical output, summary statistics, and various analytic tools, such as filtering).
- The need to replace the Latin Hypercube Sampling algorithm to improve convergence for models that rely on adequate representation of the low-probability regions of probability distributions.

Note that those types of risks and benefits generically apply to all such choices and are not limited to @RISK or the particular custom simulation implementation developed by USDA. It is important to clarify that the decision faced by USDA should not be seen as a choice among the two modeling environments.

The issues raised here are of general interest to the broader community performing and using microbial risk assessments. USDA and Food and Drug Administration risk assessors are among the leaders in this field. Given the importance of the United States as a trading partner and the potential (but as yet undemonstrated) importance of microbial risk assessments in the international food trade, their choices of modeling environments and software are influential. The influence is based on the desire for compatibility of approaches and the fact that such models and approaches will be (and have been) copied in other countries and at the international level.

Explication of the Model

At the suggestion of the committee, FSIS developed a summary (Appendix C, "Model Equations and Code") of the variables and equations used in the model. However, it is not sufficient for following the flow of information and computation in the model. The combination of explicit cell calculations and VBA-based calculations makes the flow of data difficult to follow. When viewing the spreadsheet for instance, it is not immediately clear whether data in a cell are truly constant (for example, a cell containing the value 300.33) or are results of a VBA calculation and therefore may change at any time. For a model with this level of complexity, more attention to the ability to document the mathematical and computational basis of the model is required.

Appendix C is a good beginning but is of limited usefulness, largely because of its use of spreadsheet cell references and its lack of a central, cross-referenced list of all variables. For each variable, the list should include its name or symbol, a description of the quantity, its units, its intended use as in input for other variables, a reference to or summary of its empirical justification, and its value or distribution or equation. The documentation should also be explicit about whether the variables are assumed to be mutually independent, correlated, or otherwise dependent.

Therefore the committee recommends that the authors review the choice of modeling environments (particularly the use of spreadsheets), simulation engines, and other implementation elements in light of all the benefits, risks, and costs associated with the many alternatives available to perform the modeling function. The choice should be based on explicit consideration of the diverse goals of the risk-assessment process both for a particular application and also as a general matter of policy support in domestic and international decision-making, and the choice should be defended in the text of the assessment.

The final risk assessment should include an explicit list of all the variables and equations that constitute the model. This recommendation is coupled with the need to find a modeling environment that is compatible with the complexity of the model and the communication and documentation issues that are inherent in preparing and presenting such a model.

JUSTIFICATION OF MODELING ASSUMPTIONS

This section reviews the reasonableness of the justifications offered in the draft assessment for the distributions and dependencies used in the Monte Carlo simulation. This chapter of the draft does not discuss the justification of the *form of the mathematical model* (such as the level of abstraction, which variables are included in the model, and which equations tie them together). Other chapters address that topic and the relevant underlying science about E. coli contamination and disease etiology.

Distribution Shapes

To use Monte Carlo simulation, an analyst is required to specify input probability distributions precisely. The difficulties in developing and justifying input distributions are well known in the field of risk analysis and have received much attention (Finley et al., 1994; Haimes et al., 1994). Although there is a considerable literature on the subject of estimating probability distributions from empirical data (Cullen and Frey, 1999; Morgan and Henrion, 1990), standard statistical approaches are of little practical value when data are sparse. In almost all risk assessments, analysts typically have little empirical evidence to support the distributions they select as inputs. As a result, the analyses usually require assumptions that cannot be completely justified by an appeal to the evidence. The consequences may be substantial because the results of probabilistic risk analyses can sometimes be sensitive to the choice of distributions used as inputs, and this sensitivity is usually strongest for the tail probabilities where risk assessments often focus their attention (Bukowski et al., 1995).

In the draft risk assessment, several methods were used for selecting the (marginal) distributions for the simulation. Outside reviewer Edmund Crouch argues (in Appendix D of this report) that several distribution choices are not scientifically justified, but his criticism may be the result of inconsistency in the modeling decisions made by the development team and, perhaps more important, of a lack of transparency in their documentation of the criteria they used for selecting distributions. The use of several criteria makes the documentation hard to evaluate. Even though using diverse strategies and criteria would not necessarily lead to discrepancies in the assessment, it seems desirable to have a clearly articulated and coherent strategy for selecting the marginal distributions.

The committee notes that no distribution selection strategy is free of all controversy. The following subsections describe the most important criticisms of each approach used by the FSIS development team. By using several strategies and not justifying the choice of one over another in any context, the draft risk assessment exposes itself to all these criticisms.

Traditional or Convenient Distributions

Sometimes data for variables in the model were fitted to a traditional or mathematically convenient distribution shape. For instance, the within-herd prevalence distribution was taken to be exponential because it conveniently had a single parameter, and, when fitted to data by the method of moments (a mathematical means of deriving the population distribution of a variable on the basis of a sample), the fit was deemed adequate. In other cases, uniform distributions were selected for second-order distributions. There is little or no justification for such choices. Whenever distributions are selected or justified on grounds that appeal to mathematical convenience, this fact must be clearly acknowledged. It could be accomplished, for example, by placing all such model choices in one place in the documentation so that the choices and their inherent consequences in the assessment could be considered together.

Empirical Distribution Functions

In several cases, empirical distributions were used as inputs in the draft model. Many analysts consider empirical distributions as the best possible representations of variability because they let the available data "speak for themselves." If all variables were treated this way, the Monte Carlo simulation would amount to a permutation study of the raw data. Risk analysts often prefer that approach because it does not require them to make assumptions about the distribution shapes or to fit distributions to data; the data *are* the distributions. The approach relies strongly on an assumption of the representativeness of the data; if the sample data are not an adequate characterization of the underlying distribution from which they were sampled, the assessment could be misled.

Cullen and Frey (1999) review strategies for computing empirical distributions from data. When data are abundant, this approach can yield an excellent characterization of the patterns of variability. When data are sparse, the characterization may still be reasonably good, depending on whether the data happen to be representative of their underlying distribution. Although the impact of sampling error obviously is increasingly important as sample size decreases, its effect is usually not incorporated into or accounted for with an empirical distribution. The primary concern about using empirical distributions as inputs in a risk assessment is that they will tend to underestimate tail probabilities. After all, unless the original sampling is very thorough and makes a special effort to observe extreme values, it is likely that, for instance, the largest value of a variable that was observed in a limited sample will actually be the largest possible value of the variable. Moreover, because distribution tails are characterized by low probabilities, sampling will typically produce few observations in the tails. Consequently, the analyst's ability to fashion good estimates of tail probabilities will be hampered if the sample is small. That is especially troublesome because it is often the tails that are of primary concern in a risk analysis focusing on extreme events that lead to disease. It is thus desirable for modelers to take pains to consider the possibilities of values outside the observed range for all variables for which empirical distributions are used.

Maximum Entropy

Some distribution selections in the FSIS draft risk assessment seem to have been based on appeals to the maximum entropy criterion, which states that when one has only partial information about possible outcomes, one should exploit the available information to the extent practicable and impose as few assumptions as possible on the missing information (Grandy and Schick, 1991; Jaynes, 1957; Lee and Wright, 1994; Levine and Tribus, 1976; Tilwari and Hobbie, 1976). The use of maximum entropy in selecting input distributions for Monte Carlo analysis is superior to naive conjecture and is considered by many to be the state of the art. The maximum entropy criterion is controversial, however. Among several criticisms, perhaps the most serious is that the model of uncertainty it uses is inconsistent through changes of scale. For instance, suppose that all one knows about a particular positive variable A is its range. The maximum entropy criterion would suggest using a uniform distribution over this range to represent the state of knowledge. Now consider the related variable A^2. If all that is known about A is its range, then surely all that is known about A^2 is its range, which is just the interval between (left bound of A)^2 and (right bound of A)^2. That means that one should pick another uniform distribution to model A^2, too. But given the uniform distribution for A, one can compute the distribution it implies for A^2, and this is not uniform over the squared range. Similar problems occur when log and other transformations are used or when a variable is arithmetically combined with other variables. The inconsistencies mean that analysts must arbitrarily pick a scale on which to express their uncertainty and resist comparing it across different scales.

Expert Elicitation

Formal expert elicitation does not appear to have been used explicitly in the draft model, but the committee suggests that it could be judiciously applied in some circumstances (notably in the Preparation Module) where single or small numbers of observations are extrapolated to the entire population.

There are various approaches to eliciting information about input variables from experts or other knowledgeable persons. They range from simply asking them in informal and uncontrolled settings to using elaborate formal schemes (Cooke, 1991; Meyer and Booker, 1991; Morgan and Henrion, 1990; Warren-Hicks and Moore, 1998). Formal elicitation schemes can often be expensive. It might be reasonable to let experts define the shapes of input distributions subjectively, but this is not always a workable strategy and, when experts disagree, it can lead to even more controversy about the inputs. In the final analysis, the committee believes that there are circumstances in which it would be appropriate to solicit expert opinion regarding point estimates and distributions and that, if found useful, such information should be documented in the text and used in the model until data become available.

Dependencies

It appears that most of the variables in the FSIS draft risk assessment are assumed to be mutually independent. Overall, the draft is practically silent on the potential for input variables to be dependent. Although such assumptions make the computation for a model substantially easier, their justification, whether theoretical or empirical, is lacking. For instance, average carcass weight may be correlated with within-feedlot prevalence (Dargatz et al., 1997). Other candidates for dependence include any variables describing consumer behavior and preferences that may share a risk factor, such as age, ethnicity, sex, or health status.

In the interest of discovering particularly high-risk scenarios, the modelers should review the list of model inputs for pairs or triplets of inputs that are intuitively likely to be dependent. The review could be based on data (perhaps rarely), reasoning regarding a common cause, or where the variables may be expected to be affected by a common general risk factor (knowledge of preparer regarding appropriate food handling or preparation practices) that is otherwise important in the assessment (such as serving size, frequency of consumption of raw ground beef, or the age of the consumer). The committee recognizes that finding concrete evidence for individual important variables is difficult; evidence of the dependence structure of two or more variables will certainly be more rare. An explicit model of such dependence may not be feasible, but the effect of plausible dependence scenarios should be considered on a case-by-case basis and presumably prioritized through causal reasoning of the plausibility of the dependence relationships. This will assist in better characterizing the potential for high-risk scenarios and may help to explain higher proportions of attributable risk to particular exposure pathways. In addition, explicit reference to the plausibility of key variable dependencies (even if difficult to quantify) is useful information for risk-management and data-collection priority-setting.

Therefore the committee recommends that the final risk assessment should address the potential for input-variable dependence in the model, based on causal reasoning and other evidence of such relationships. For potentially important dependencies, a sensitivity analysis should be performed to evaluate the nature and magnitude of the potential dependence structure.

Seasonality

The draft pays considerable attention to assumptions regarding the seasonal pattern of on-farm prevalence. As mentioned in Chapter 2 and Appendix D of this report, the data cited as justification for modeling seasonality in prevalence do not actually provide evidence of such seasonality. In face-to-face meetings, analysts of the development team suggest that the best evidence comes from studies conducted outside the United States; they were omitted out of relevance concerns, but the omission leaves the assertion about seasonality essentially unsupported. The relevance concerns about foreign studies should be resolved and documented so that justification for seasonality assumptions is clarified.

Therefore the committee recommends that the authors should reconsider the evidence of and the approach for inferring seasonality in on-farm prevalence, including the potential for using data from outside the United States. Evidence of seasonality might also be sought in the upper tails of the internal or external pathogen load among *E. coli* O157:H7 -positive animals. That may have a stronger effect (by several orders of magnitude) than simple variations in prevalence on the number of contaminated ground-beef patties. The committee recognizes that, given the substantial uncertainty associated with other important quantities in the model that affect prevalence downstream, further refinement of the exact pattern of on-farm seasonality may not have high priority.

OVERALL MODEL UNCERTAINTY AND RELIABILITY

It appears that several of the methods used in developing the draft risk assessment may tend to understate uncertainty. That would typically be considered disadvantageous, if not dangerous, in risk analyses. There are several ways this happens: incomplete reconstruction of statistical regressions, overreliance on empirical distributions, use of means other than raw data, and modeling of sampling variation without representing the underlying uncertainty arising from measurement error. Each of those is discussed below.

Uncertainty Encoded in Regressions Not Reconstructed

The draft makes use of several regression analyses, but in doing so it seems to have not fully reconstructed the uncertainty in the relationship among the random variables in the original data sets. For instance, in Equation 3.28 (described on p. 80 of the draft and p. 196 of Appendix C), constants are used to transform temperature linearly into *E. coli* generation time. The coefficients of the linear scaling appear to be regression parameters (Marks et al., 1998), but the regression model has not been used to re-express the uncertainty in the predicted variable. Instead, the linear scaling is the prediction of the *mean* value of generation time expected, given a particular temperature. That approach does not reconstruct even the scatter of the original data, much less account for sampling uncertainty. Similar applications of slope and intercept values are made in the equations for calculating the lag period for *E. coli* O157:H7 for a specific step of handling or storage (Equation 3.27) and the maximum population density of the pathogen in ground beef (Equation 3.29).

Overreliance on Empirical Distributions

The fact that empirical distributions typically underestimate the probabilities of values in distribution tails is a straightforward result of the reality that, given any limited random sample, the chance of ever observing the rare events in the tails is low. The authors seem to place too much credence in distributions that are based on remarkably few data points. In the case of Equation 3.11.1, described on p. 179 of Appendix C, the distribution of the number of bacteria per square centimeter of carcass surface area is specified from only four points. No accounting is made of the sampling error or measurement error implied by that small number. The problem is essentially the same as one encounters when using only a single study in a scientific review. Because of the importance of distribution tails, the problem is also similar to using the *observed* maximum of a sample as the *theoretical* maximum of a random variable.

Modelers need to account for sampling error to see beyond the limited data available. In principle, Kolmogorov-Smirnov confidence intervals could be computed that characterize the sampling uncertainty about the distribution as a whole, assuming that the samples were independent and identically distributed. In any case, the uncertainty about distribution shape should be explicitly and quantitatively characterized. Doing so will allow analysts to revisit the choice of distribution shape in later sensitivity and robustness studies.

Use of Averages

At many points in the *E. coli* assessment, the modelers use *average* values of variables rather than a distribution of various quantities. An average does not capture variability; it erases it. Consequently, averages are of little use in a risk assessment, where one of the primary concerns is to account for variability in the system. In the case of some variables, a distribution is used, but it is a distribution of values that turn out to be averages over one or more dimensions. In such cases, the distributions represent only part of the true variability of the underlying variable.

Untenably Precise Submodels

The overall assessment will underestimate uncertainty if it is composed of submodels that underestimate the uncertainties in the variables they are used to model. One example in the draft is the model of cooking loss. Figure 3-25 on p. 88 in the draft risk assessment depicts the modeled frequency distribution of log reductions in *E. coli* abundance caused from cooking. It also depicts the uncertainty about this distribution by displaying 20 realizations of the distribution. It seems implausible that the true distribution of reductions, whatever it is, has the multimodality that this figure shows. The problem is not the "bumpiness" of the distribution itself, but the fact that the same bumpiness persists in all the realizations of the distribution—that is, the bumpiness is stronger than the overall uncertainty about the distribution.

As explained in Appendix D of the FSIS draft ("Modeling Issues"), the origin of the multimodality can be traced to the cooking-temperature data on which the model of log reductions was based. Each distribution of the ensemble displayed in the figure is based on integrating (apparently, actually a *stochastic mixture* of) nine distributions representing the effect of cooking with different pretreatments. A mixture model would be appropriate if the analysts knew the relative frequencies of the various pretreatments in homes and institutions. However, it seems that the mixture in this case is used to represent model uncertainty rather than the variability among kitchens.

For each pretreatment, a regression is computed from 18 points (six replicates at each of three cooking temperatures), and the *mean* reduction is taken from the regression line. That seems to be the real reason that the uncertainty in the distribution of log reductions is so small. The mean reduction does not seem entirely relevant. It is the outliers of the distribution (small reductions) that are likely to induce illness. It seems that the modelers strive to make their assessment consistent with the observed data but sacrificed the reliability of their results to do so.

As noted in Appendix D of the FSIS draft, the bumpiness of the distribution can be traced finally to the preferences for round numbers in the values reported for final cooking temperature on the Fahrenheit scale (for example, 150°F rather than 153°F). It seems clear that the modality is completely artifactual. That is not at all a criticism of the original data—it is how the survey turned out. However, that the bumpiness persisted through the many transformations made on the data suggests that the true scope of their inherent uncertainty was never fully recognized. In summary, the original data, with their multimodality, seem fine; what is insufficient is the breadth of uncertainty about the final distribution of log reductions.

The committee notes that if the modelers had simply smoothed the distribution before computing and displaying the uncertainty about it, the problem might never have been noticed. Their openness in portraying the details of this particular variable and the data it was based on demonstrates the utility of transparency in presentation.

Inappropriate Use of Bayesian Formulations

The committee suspects that the use of beta distributions in Equation 3.10.1, described on p. 177 of Appendix C of the FSIS draft, exemplifies another way in which the uncertainty present in the system is underestimated in the draft model. That equation defines the random variable TR (transformation ratio), which is the multiplier of the *E. coli* prevalence in cattle that predicts the prevalence in carcasses. Data collected from four slaughter plants during July and August (Elder et al., 2000) suggest that TR is about 160%. (The ratio is larger than 1 presumably as a result of cross contamination during dehiding.) The counts actually reported were 91 of 307 cattle and 148 of 312 carcasses being contaminated. The authors explain that the beta distributions are used to model the uncertainty about TR. The beta distributions arise in this context from a simple Bayesian updating argument about frequency estimates. However, the specified beta distributions have extremely small variances; both are less than 0.001. Given the ordinary fluctuations one might anticipate from day to day and across slaughter plants, it seems entirely unreasonable to expect that such distributions could be realistic models of the contaminated fractions of cattle or carcasses. Because the numerator and denominator in Equation 3.10.1 are combined under an (unsupported) assumption of independence, the quotient has a very small variance, which suggests that the ultimate *TR* has little uncertainty.

Potentially Dominant Model Uncertainties

Model uncertainty is a class of uncertainty that pertains to the adequacy of a model's representation of reality. Strictly on the basis of qualitative judgment, the committee suggests that the following general model uncertainties may dominate:

• *The ability to define an appropriate output or set of outputs from the on-farm module that is adequately correlated with the level of risk to the ground-beef supply.* As described in the review of the Production Module (Chapter 3 of this report), prevalence estimates can vary considerably with detection method, type, and definition (for example, cattle with 1 or more EHEC on the entire surface or in the entire gut). It is intuitively reasonable to suggest that the number and relative proportion of animals with very high bacterial loads will dominate the overall contamination level in the combo bin, given the fact that the contamination (through pooling in the combo bins and grinders) is proportional to the total across many individual contributions. Given the expectation of logarithmic variability in pathogen loads, the highest-shedding animals will contribute more bacteria (by a factor of several powers of 10) whenever there is a transfer to the carcass surface. Conversely, the animal with an *average burden* may contribute comparably little.

• *The ability to represent the transfer of organisms from the hide or gut of the animal to the carcass surface and the relationship between measurements of cell density on the carcass surface and the amount on trim that becomes ground beef.*

• *The ability to represent the potential for reservoirs of contamination in a slaughter plant and for cross contamination of carcasses.* The potential pathways and reservoirs of contamination in a slaughter plant are numerous, complex, and likely to be dynamically changing, even if measured. The use of indicator organisms should be reconsidered for their ability to track the sources and extent of fecal contamination in the plant. Without a drastic change in the approach to data gathering and modeling, this part of the model will remain a "black box." Attempts to model its internal mechanisms may be misguided until appropriate data are made available to the modelers.

- *The prevalence of exposure to uncooked ground beef.* This variable will be inherently difficult to estimate because of the uncommon nature of the exposure and the response bias associated with its estimation from surveys or other methods. However, it could be important because there may be a relatively high probability of illness associated with the pathway compared with a cooked product.

- *The extent of the exposure that occurs through cross contamination.* The committee recognizes that there are no examples of risk-assessment modules that could adequately describe the potential for risk associated with cross contamination during food preparation. Even an emerging experimental database that focuses on cross contamination is unlikely to support such a model in sufficient detail to form predictions of illness through this complex pathway in the near future. This remains a major methodologic hurdle in microbiologic risk assessment.

- *The dose-response relationship for EHEC.* Despite the committee's suggestion that a *Shigella* species may constitute an adequate surrogate for the best estimate of the dose-response function, there remains broad uncertainty associated with this representation and even with the characterization of the dose-response function for *Shigella* itself. While it may ultimately be possible to narrow the uncertainty envelope used in the draft risk assessment, large uncertainties will remain regarding the dose that corresponds to a given probability of illness.

Use of Undefined Variables

One of the features of an Excel spreadsheet is the automatic initialization (to zero) of variables that are not otherwise explicitly defined. Automatic initialization is regarded as a feature of convenience when beginning a model, but can become a serious hindrance as the model develops. Appendix D, which contains comments on the model presented to the committee by outside reviewer Edmund Crouch, cites specific examples where references were found to undefined cells in the draft model spreadsheet. Some of these cells had been given a "hatched" format, presumably to indicate that the values were not available. Because of automatic initialization, Excel regarded the undefined cells as zeros. Although this may turn out to be the correct value to use for these particular variables, **the committee suggests that the final risk assessment explicitly define all variables and constants to be used in the model, simply as a matter of good modeling practice.**

Unit Conformance

Experience with complex assessments has shown that profound errors can arise from simple or careless mistakes in units (Isbell et al., 1999). It is thus important that quantities to be added, subtracted, or compared for magnitude have conforming units; and quantities to be used as exponents or powers or the arguments of logarithms be dimensionless (Hart, 1995).

The FSIS draft report's Appendix C—a partial list of the model equations and code—contains some but not all of the information needed to check unit conformance. The committee was thus unable to conduct a rigorous review of the dimensions and units of the equations and variables used in the draft model. It suggests that the final model's mathematical expressions be checked for dimensional soundness and the input quantities be checked for unit conformity with the variables in the expression.

Overall Assessment of Model Reliability

The committee believes that a forthright and comprehensive characterization of the uncertainty in the assessment would show the overall model uncertainty to be very large (much larger than suggested by the Risk Characterization chapter of the draft), even after anchoring. It may be that the uncertainty is so large as to appear to overwhelm any quantitative predictions based on the assessment. But even if that is so, the authors should not shy away from being as forthright and comprehensive as possible. Large uncertainty itself does not preclude useful applications of an assessment. But underestimated uncertainty can threaten the credibility of an assessment and lead to unwarranted confidence on the part of decision-makers regarding the response of the system being modeled to simulated mitigations.

Therefore the committee recommends that the final report clearly describe the magnitude of model uncertainty related to key modules in the risk assessment and include strategies for reducing the uncertainty, if they exist.

REFERENCES

Brand KP, Small MJ. 1995. Updating uncertainty in an integrated risk assessment: Conceptual framework and methods. Risk Analysis 15(6):719–731.

Bukowski J, Korn L, Wartenberg D. 1995. Correlated inputs in quantitative risk assessment: The effects of distributional shape. Risk Analysis 15:215–219.

Burmaster DE, Anderson PD. 1994. Principles of good practice for the use of Monte Carlo techniques in human health and ecological risk assessments. Risk Analysis 14:477–481.

Cassin MH, Lammerding AM, Todd EC, Ross W, McColl RS. 1998. Quantitative risk assessment of *Escherichia coli* O157:H7 in ground beef hamburgers. International Journal of Food Microbiology 41:21–44.

Cooke RM. 1991. Experts in Uncertainty. Cambridge: Oxford University Press.

Cullen AC, Frey HC. 1999. Probabilistic Techniques in Exposure Assessment: A Handbook for Dealing with Variability and Uncertainty in Models and Inputs. New York: Plenum Press.

Dargatz DA, Wells SJ, Thomas LA, Hancock DD, Garber LP. 1997. Factors associated with the presence of *Escherichia coli* O157 in feces in feedlot cattle. Journal of Food Protection 60:466–470.

DeWaal CS, Barlow K, Alderton L, Jacobson MF. 2001. Outbreak Alert! Closing the Gaps in Our Federal Food Safety Net. Washington, DC: Center for Science in the Public Health Interest. October.

Dilks DW, Canale RP, Meier PG. 1992. Development of a Bayesian Monte Carlo method for determining water quality model uncertainty. Ecological Modeling 62:149–162.

Elder RO, Keen JE, Siragusa GR, Barkocy-Gallagher GA, Koomaraie M, Laegreid WW. 2000. Correlation of enterohemorrhagic *E. coli* O157 prevalence in feces, hides, and carcasses of beef cattle during processing. Proceedings of the National Academy of Sciences 97(7):2999–3003.

Finley B, Proctor D, Scott P, Harrington N, Pasutenbach D, Price P. 1994. Recommended distributions for exposure factors frequently used in health risk assessment. Risk Analysis 14:533–553.

Gelman A, Carlin JB, Stern HS, Rubin DB. 1995. Bayesian Data Analysis. London: Chapman and Hall.

Grandy WT Jr, Schick LH. 1991. Maximum Entropy and Bayesian Methods. Dordrecht: Kluwer Academic Publishers.

Green, EJ, MacFarlane DW, Valentine HT. 2000. Bayesian synthesis for quantifying uncertainty in predictions from process models. Tree Physiology 20:415–419.

Haimes YY, Barry T, Lambert JH. 1994. When and how can you specify a probability distribution when you don't know much? Risk Analysis 14:661–706.

Hart GW. 1995. Multidimensional Analysis: Algebras and Systems for Science and Engineering. New York: Springer Verlag.

Isbell D, Hardin M, Underwood J. 1999. Mars Climate Orbiter team finds likely cause of loss. Mars Climate Orbiter/Mars Polar Lander News & Status Release 99-113 (dated September 30, 1999) http://mars.jpl.nasa.gov/msp98/news/mco990930.html.

Jaynes ET. 1957. Information theory and statistical mechanics. Physical Review 106:620–630.

Kassenborg H, Hedberg C, Hoekstra M, Evans MC, Chin AE, Marcus R, Vugia D, Smith K, Desai S, Slutsker L, Griffin P, and the FoodNet Working Group. 2001. Farm visits and undercooked hamburgers as major risk factors for sporadic *Escherichia coli* O157:H7 infections—Data from a case-control study in five FoodNet sites. Manuscript in preparation.

Lee RC, Wright WE. 1994. Development of human exposure-factor distributions using maximum-entropy inference. Journal of Exposure Analysis and Environmental Epidemiology 4:329–341.

Levine RD, Tribus M. 1976. The Maximum Entropy Formalism. Cambridge: MIT Press.

Marks HM, Coleman ME, Lin CTJ, Roberts T. 1998. Topics in risk assessment: Dynamic flow tree process. Risk Analysis 18:309–328.

Meyer MA, Booker JM. 1991. Eliciting and Analyzing Expert Judgment: A Practical Guide. New York: Academic Press.

Morgan MG, Henrion M. 1990. Uncertainty: A Guide to Dealing with Uncertainty in Quantitative Risk and Policy Analysis. Cambridge: Cambridge University Press.

Nauta MJ, Evers EG, Takumi K, Havelaar AH. 2001. Risk assessment of Shiga-toxin producing *Escherichia coli* O157 in steak tartare in the Netherlands. Rijksinstituut voor Volksgezondheid en Milieu (RIVM). Report 257851 003.

Shinagawa K. 1997. Correspondence and problem for enterohemorrhagic *E. coli* O157 outbreak in Morioka city, Iwate. Koshu Eisei Kenkyu 46:104–112.

Small MJ, Fischbeck PS. 1999. False precision in Bayesian updating with incomplete models. Journal of Human and Ecological Risk Assessment 5(2):291–304.

Tilwari JL, Hobbie JE. 1976. Random differential equations as models of ecosystems. II. Initial condition and parameter specification in terms of maximum entropy distributions. Mathematical Biosciences 31:37–53.

Warren-Hicks WJ, Moore DRJ. 1998. Uncertainty Analysis in Ecological Risk Assessment. Pensacola, FL.: SETAC Press, Chapter 3.

Appendix A

Agendas of Public Meetings Held by the Committee on the Review of the USDA *E. coli* O157:H7 Farm-to-Table Risk Assessment

FIRST PUBLIC MEETING

Monday, September 24, 2001
Room 2004, The Foundry Building
Washington, D.C.
Presentations

- **Sponsor's charge to the committee**
  I. Kaye Wachsmuth PhD
  United States Department of Agriculture (USDA),
  Food Safety and Inspection Service (FSIS)
  Deputy Administrator, FSIS, Office of Public Health and Science

- **USDA-FSIS *E. coli* risk assessment model**
  Wayne D. Schlosser, DVM; Eric D. Ebel, DVM; Kathleen Orloski, DVM
  USDA, FSIS, Office of Public Health and Science, Risk Assessment Division

SECOND PUBLIC MEETING

Monday, December 17, 2001
Board Room, NAS Building
Washington, D.C.

Presentations

- **Comments on USDA-FSIS draft risk assessment of the public health impact of *Escherichia coli* O157:H7 in ground beef**
  Anna M. Lammerding, PhD
  Chief, Microbial Food Safety Risk Assessment
  Health Canada, Laboratory Centre for Foodborne Zoonoses
  Guelph, Ontario

- **Comments on the review of the USDA-FSIS *E. coli* O157:H7 farm-to-table process risk assessment**
  Edmund A.C. Crouch, PhD
  Senior Scientist
  Cambridge Environmental Inc.
  Cambridge, Massachusetts

- Public input and discussion among session participants.

Appendix B

Additional Comments

The body of this report contains the principal comments of the committee regarding the content of the draft US Department of Agriculture *E. coli* O157:H7 risk assessment. This appendix contains a number of additional comments regarding citations, typographic errors, and the like that the committee wishes to bring to the attention of the draft's authors. The comments are listed by page number.

Page 12: In the list of outputs of the Production Module, insert the words "use in manufacturing" (or a comparable descriptive phrase) after the word "for" in "prior to slaughter for ground beef."

Page 25: The study by Brackett (not Brachett) et al. (1994) was of decontamination of meat cuts, not carcasses as implied.

Page 32: The word "proportion" may be better than the word "share" in describing amounts of imported and domestic ground beef consumed, which could explain the findings.

Page 33: "Test sensitivity is a complex parameter that incorporates variability in sample collection and handling and in the biological properties of the sample": the meaning of the statement is unclear. It should simply be stated that sample variability may affect apparent test sensitivity.

Page 33: "The slaughter plant intake segment considers the effect of clustering cattle as they enter the slaughter plant": this would apply to cows and bulls, which may have different sources and be commingled; steers and heifers from feedlots, however, are not mixed with cattle from other groups.

Page 39: "Although evidence is limited, it suggests that dairy cow-calf herds are similar with respect to *E. coli* O157:H7": it is not clear what regarding O157:H7 is similar.

Page 51: "Five studies provide evidence on apparent within-feedlot": insert the word "prevalence" after that phrase.

Page 51: "... this protocol is assumed to be 100% sensitive": a reason should be provided for this assumption.

Page 53: The age of breeding cattle is more likely 3, instead of 2, years; most feedlot cattle should be 1–2 years old.

Page 56: Truckloads of cattle from different feedlots are not usually mixed at slaughter.

Page 65: The draft risk assessment cites Sheridan et al. (1992) as having identified such equipment as knives, gloves, and aprons as reservoirs of bacteria in the slaughterhouse. That is correct, but the reference also indicates that "the level of contamination varied with different cuts of meat," which may affect the extent of contamination of trim. There is also a typographic error in the citation: *Meat Science* 32:185–194, rather than 32:155–164.

Page 66: Contrary to what is stated in the draft, no "excess fat is trimmed away from each side" of the carcass at splitting (before washing), although blood-soiled tissue may be trimmed.

Page 67: The draft asserts that distilled water and chlorine are occasionally sprayed on carcasses in chillers (Step 6). Carcasses are spray-chilled with water but not with distilled water or chlorine (which causes corrosion). Lactic acid may be in the initial stages of finding some use in this application.

Page 67: "FSIS regulations require chilling deep muscle (6 inches) to 10.0°C (50.0°F) within 24 hours and 7.2°C (45.0°F) within 36 hours (NACMCF, 1993)": this may be done in practice but to the committee's knowledge, is not required by the Food Safety and Inspection Service; if it is, a more direct reference should be provided.

Page 67: "Dorsa (1997) found a 1.2 log CFU/cm^2 increase in *E. coli* O157:H7 on carcasses stored for 2 days in the chiller at 5.0°C (41.0°F)": It appears that the correct reference may be Dorsa et al. (1997), not Dorsa (1997). Instead of carcasses, the study evaluated inoculated beef-carcass tissue samples that were decontaminated and packaged, thus simulating retail products rather than carcasses. In addition, it is questionable whether *E. coli* O157:H7 would grow at 5°C.

Page 68: "Prasai et al. (1995) found no difference in concentrations of *E. coli* O157:H7 between hot deboning and cold deboning": it appears that the Prasai et al. (1995) reference listed does not deal with *E. coli* O157:H7 or hot or cold deboning.

Page 70: The carcass surface areas estimated to end up in ground beef seem high (75–90%; citing McAloon, 1999), given that much of the external carcass surface fat is trimmed away during fabrication and is used in rendering. One major concern is the issue of estimating surface area of trim, considering the extensive cutting that takes place during fabrication.

Page 77: Combo bins contain trim, not ground beef.

Page 77: Newer data may be available for ground-beef proportions used at retail and in hotels, restaurants, and institutions (HRI); retail grinding may have decreased. The draft apparently does not, but should, consider coarse ground-beef chubs.

Page 79/81: Palumbo (1997), which is cited in the text, is not in the reference list.

Page 82, 83: Citations of the unpublished Vose 1999 manuscript should be updated to a published reference if at all possible.

Page 95: The report needs to specify how combinatorial mathematics was used to compute the convolutions instead of Monte Carlo simulation.

Page 100: The Gill (1996) reference may be incorrectly listed.

Page 124: MPN is not CFU. Most probable number and colony forming units are measures of microbial density measured differently.

Page 131: Footnote 2 refers to Table 5-1, but the data appear to be in Table 5-2.

Page 142: The draft report's correlation analysis states that "the size of the *E. coli* O157:H7-contaminated carcass surface was the only factor correlated (coefficient = 0.33) with the number of *E. coli* O157:H7 organisms in steer/heifer combo bins (Table 5-3)." It should be noted that there is no evidence (and it is probably impossible to obtain evidence) on the size of the area of a carcass that is contaminated. In addition, contamination is not expected to occur uniformly on a given carcass area (whatever the area); contamination usually occurs as clumps of cells in microscopic environments.

Page 166: How is it possible that deterministic values "come from a distribution" but "do not change as a result of Monte Carlo iteration"?

Page 170: Here and elsewhere in Appendix C there are some apparent inconsistencies in the definition of the term *deterministic*. For instance, in Equation 3.3, how can Hsens be deterministic if one of the variables used to calculate it— p_i —is stochastic?

Page 183: The last word in the description of Equation 3.15 should be "evisceration" rather than "dehiding."

Page 206: Here and elsewhere in Appendix C, what does it mean when the space reserved to declare a variable as deterministic or stochastic is left blank?

Appendix D, page 3: Minus signs, rather than parentheses, should be used to denote negative values for consistency with the rest of the draft.

The temperature scale (Celsius) used in the regression should be mentioned. The words *incorporating* and *ste-y* should be defined or explained in the text.

REFERENCES FROM THE DRAFT RISK ASSESSMENT THAT NEED TO BE CORRECTED

Cassin MH, Lammerding AM, Todd EC, Ross W, McColl RS. 1998. Quantitative risk assessment of *Escherichia coli* O157:H7 in ground beef hamburgers. International Journal of Food Microbiology 41:21–44.

Codex Alimentarius Commission. 1999. Principles and Guidelines for the Conduct of Microbiological Risk Assessment. CAC/GL-30. Food and Agricultural Organization of the United Nations.

FDA/USDA 2001. Draft Assessment of the Relative Risk to Public Health from Foodborne *Listeria monocytogenes* Among Selected Categories of Ready-to-Eat Foods. FDA/Center for Food Safety and Applied Nutrition, USDA/Food Safety and Inspection Service, Centers for Disease Control and Prevention, January 2001. http://www.foodsafety.gov/~dms/lmrisk.html.

ILSI Risk Science Institute. 2000. Revised Framework for Microbial Risk Assessment—An ILSI Risk Science Institute Workshop report. Washington, DC: International Life Sciences Institute.

Marks HM, Coleman ME, Lin CTJ, Roberts T. 1998. Topics in risk assessment: Dynamic flow tree process. Risk Analysis 18:309–328.

Smeltzer TI, Peel B, Collins G. 1979. The role of equipment that has direct contact with the carcase in the spread of *Salmonella* in a beef abattoir. Australian Veterinary Journal 55:275–277.

WHO (World Health Institute), 1995. Application of Risk Analysis to Food Standards Issues-The report of the Joint FAO/WHO Expert Consultation, 13–17 March 1995 (WHO/FNU/FOS/95.3).

Appendix C

Committee and Staff Biographies

MICHEAL P. DOYLE, PhD (*Chair*), is the Regents Professor of Food Microbiology and director of the Center for Food Safety at the University of Georgia. Dr. Doyle is one the best-known food microbiologists in the United States, and is recognized internationally. He has conducted extensive research on foodborne pathogens—including *E. coli* O157:H7—and authored more than 200 papers and several books. He has consulted extensively with the food industry and has served in and chaired multiple committees of International Life Sciences Institute, World Health Organization, the American Society for Microbiology, the International Association for Food Protection, Institute of Food Technologists, and many other professional societies. He has been a member of the National Advisory Committee on Microbiological Criteria for Foods (1988–1990, 1994–2000) and the International Commission on Microbiological Specifications for Foods. He has also served on Institute of Medicine committees related to animal health and food safety and as a member of the Food and Nutrition Board and the Food Forum.

SCOTT FERSON, PhD, is the senior scientist and vice president at Applied Biomathematics. Dr. Ferson's research focuses on developing reliable mathematical and statistical tools for ecologic and human health risk assessments and on methods for uncertainty analysis when empirical information is sparse. He has participated in several scientific advisory panels for the US Environmental Protection Agency, National Institutes of Health, and other government agencies. Dr. Ferson has over 60 scientific publications in environmental risk analysis and uncertainty propagation and has directed the development of several commercial software packages used in environmental and ecologic risk analysis.

DALE D. HANCOCK, DVM, MS, PhD, is a professor and epidemiologist in the Field Disease Investigation Unit of the Department of Veterinary Clinical Sciences at Washington State University. Dr. Hancock is a veterinarian who has conducted extensive research into the prevalence, risk factors, and epidemiology of *E. coli* O157:H7 in cattle. As a professor at Washington State University, he teaches courses in quantitative epidemiology and public health. Dr. Hancock has published extensively, with articles appearing in many journals, including *Epidemiology and Infection, International Journal of Food Microbiology,* and *Journal of Food Protection.* He has written chapters in two recent books by the American Society for Microbiology: *Emerging Infectious Diseases of Animals* and *Escherichia coli O157:H7 and Other Shiga Toxin Producing E. coli Strains.* Dr. Hancock is a frequent invited speaker at national and international food-safety and veterinary conferences.

MYRON M. LEVINE, MD, DTPH, is the director of the internationally recognized Center for Vaccine Development at the University of Maryland School of Medicine and holds faculty appointments as professor in four departments: Medicine, Pediatrics, Epidemiology, and Microbiology and Immunology. In two of those departments, Dr. Levine is a division head: the Division of Geographic Medicine in the Department of Medicine and the Division of Infectious Diseases and Tropical Pediatrics in the Department of Pediatrics. He has been elected to many professional societies, including the Institute of Medicine, the American Epidemiological Society, and the Association for American Physicians. He has served on many international committees and is a member of the Working Group of the Global Alliance for Vaccines and Immunization. Dr. Levine has published over 413 journal articles and serves on the editorial board of the *American Journal of Epidemiology, Public Health Reviews,* and *Vaccine.*

GREG PAOLI, MASc, is the president of Decisionalysis Risk Consultants, Inc, a firm specializing in assessment, communication, and management of health risk, primarily in the field of food safety. He has served on several international panels, most recently participating in the Expert Consultations as part of the Joint Food and Agriculture Organization and World Health Organization (FAO/WHO) activities on microbial risk assessment. He serves as chair of the Food and Water Risk Specialty Group of the Society for Risk Analysis. Mr. Paoli was part of a Canadian research team that developed a quantitative risk assessment of *E. coli* O157:H7 in ground beef. He has also published extensively in risk assessment. He holds a master's degree in systems design engineering from the University of Waterloo and served as research manager at the University's Institute for Risk Research.

BARBARA J. PETERSEN, PhD, MPH, is a principal and director of the food and chemicals practice of the consulting firm Exponent. Dr. Petersen has a doctorate in biochemistry with minors in nutrition, microbial physiology, and organic chemistry. Her primary expertise is in regulatory strategy and risk assessment, including cumulative and aggregate exposure-assessment modeling. She has extensive experience in intake-assessment modeling, including overall oversight of software development for risk assessment including CALENDEX (Calendar Based Exposure Assessment), DEEM (Dietary Exposure Evaluation Model), and FARE (Food And Residue Evaluation System). Her expertise extends to database design for automated data collection and analysis and design of computerized adaptation of Monte Carlo analysis for computing the probability of exposure to food contaminants, including microbial contamination.

JOHN N. SOFOS, PhD, is a professor in the Department of Animal Sciences at Colorado State University. In addition to teaching, Dr. Sofos is a science adviser for the Food and Drug Administration at the Denver District Laboratory and a scientific coeditor of the *Journal of Food Protection*. He is well known for his studies on the microbiology of meat-processing operations, particularly at the slaughterhouse level and in relation to decontamination steps for beef carcasses, as well as the microbiology of processed-meat products and other ready-to-eat foods. He is experienced in the hazard analysis and critical control point (HACCP) food-safety assurance method. Dr. Sofos has conducted research to estimate the prevalence of *E. coli* O157:H7 in live cattle and its survivability in raw-meat products. He has published extensively in foodborne microorganisms and microbiology.

SUSAN N. SUMNER, PhD, is associate professor, department head, and extension project leader in the Department of Food Science and Technology at Virginia Polytechnic Institute and State University. Dr. Sumner earned her MS and PhD in food science-food safety from the University of Wisconsin-Madison. Before accepting her position at Virginia Polytechnic Institute, she worked for the National Food Processors' Association and was a faculty member at the University of Nebraska at Lincoln, where her work focused on beef handling and production. Her research focuses on control of pathogenic bacteria—including *Escherichia coli* O157:H7, *Salmonella*, and *Listeria monocytogenes*—to build a base of knowledge of how to control these pathogens in food-processing facilities. Her extension efforts have focused on food-safety education for the food industry. The recipient of many awards and honors, Dr. Sumner received the Educator Award in 2000 from the International Association for Food Protection. She is a member of the Experiment Station Committee on Organization and Policy Extension Committee on Organization and Policy (ESCOP/ECOP) Food Safety Taskforce and the Institute of Medicine's Food Forum. She is a member of many professional organizations and has published extensively in food safety and microbiology.

LIASON FROM THE BOARD ON HEALTH PROMOTION AND DISEASE PREVENTION

HUGH TILSON, MD, DrPH, is clinical professor of epidemiology and health policy and senior adviser to the dean of the University of North Carolina School of Public Health. He is a graduate of Washington University School of Medicine and the Harvard School of Public Health, and he is a board-certified specialist in preventive medicine. He is a former state and local public-health official and international pharmaceutical scientist, and his research contributions span public-health practice, pharmacoepidemiology, health outcomes, and policy research.

STAFF BIOGRAPHIES

ALLISON A. YATES, PhD, RD, is director of the Food and Nutrition Board (FNB) of the Institute of Medicine (IOM). Dr. Yates received a BS in dietetics and an MS in public health (nutrition) from the University of California, Los Angeles, and a PhD in nutrition from the University of California, Berkeley; she is a registered dietitian. She is a member of the American Society for Nutrition Sciences, American Society for Clinical Nutrition, American Dietetic Association, American Public Health Association, and Institute of Food Technologists. Dr. Yates served as a member of the FNB Committee on Military Nutrition Research before assuming her position at IOM in 1994. Most recently, Dr. Yates was professor of foods and nutrition and dean of the College of Health and Human Sciences at the University of Southern Mississippi.

ROSE MARIE MARTINEZ, ScD, is director of the Institute of Medicine Board on Health Promotion and Disease Prevention. Before joining IOM, she was a senior health researcher at Mathematica Policy Research, where she conducted research on the impact of health-system change on the public-health infrastructure, access to care for vulnerable populations, managed care, and the health-care workforce. Dr. Martinez is a former assistant director for health financing and policy with the US General Accounting Office, where she directed evaluations and policy analysis in national and public-health issues. Dr. Martinez received her doctorate from the Johns Hopkins School of Hygiene and Public Health.

DAVID A. BUTLER, PhD, is a senior program officer in the Institute of Medicine Board on Health Promotion and Disease Prevention. He received a BS and MS in engineering from the University of Rochester and a PhD in public policy analysis from Carnegie Mellon University. Before joining IOM, Dr. Butler served as an analyst for the US Congress Office of Technology Assessment and was Research Associate in the Department of Environmental Health at the Harvard School of Public Health. He has directed several National Academies' studies on environmental health and risk assessment topics, including those that resulted in the reports *Veterans and Agent Orange: Update 1998*, *Veterans and Agent Orange: Update 2000*, and *Clearing the Air: Asthma and Indoor Air Exposures*.

RICARDO A. MOLINS, PhD, is a senior program officer in the Institute of Medicine, Food and Nutrition Board. He received a BS, a MS, and a PhD in food science from Iowa State University. Before joining the IOM, Dr. Molins was assistant and associate professor of food microbiology with the Iowa State University Meat Export Research Center. He has also worked for several international organizations, including the United Nations Industrial Development Organization and, more recently, the International Atomic Energy Agency, in Vienna, Austria, in food safety microbiology, food irradiation, and the HACCP method. He has conducted research on microbial-decontamination methods for meat products, mechanism of action of antimicrobials in foods, and food irradiation. He is a reviewer for the *Journal of Food Protection* and has published two books and more than 50 refereed journal papers. He is study director for the Food Chemicals Codex and for the Review of the Use of Scientific Criteria and Performance Standards for Safe Food.

JENNIFER A. COHEN is a research associate in the Institute of Medicine Board on Health Promotion and Disease Prevention. She received her undergraduate degree in art history from the University of Maryland. She has also been involved with the IOM committees that produced *Organ Procurement and Transplantation; Clearing the Air: Asthma and Indoor Air Exposures; Veterans and Agent Orange: Herbicide/Dioxin Exposure and Type 2 Diabetes; Veterans and Agent Orange: Update 2000;* and *Veterans and Agent Orange: Herbicide/Dioxin Exposure and Acute Myelogenous Leukemia in the Children of Vietnam Veterans*.

ANNA B. STATON, MPA, is a research assistant in the Institute of Medicine Board on Health Promotion and Disease Prevention. Ms. Staton joined IOM in December 1999 and has worked with the committees that produced *No Time to Lose: Getting More from HIV Prevention* and *Agent Orange Update: 2000*. Before joining IOM, she worked at the Baltimore Women's Health Study. Ms. Staton graduated from the University of Maryland Baltimore County with a BA in visual arts (major) and women's studies (minor). She earned her master's of public administration degree in nonprofit management at the George Washington University School of Business and Public Management.

ELIZABETH J. ALBRIGO is a project assistant in the Institute of Medicine Board on Health Promotion and Disease Prevention. She received her undergraduate degree in psychology from the Virginia Polytechnic Institute and State University. She is currently involved with the IOM Committee on Damp Indoor Spaces and Health and Committee on the Assessment of Wartime Exposure to Herbicides in Vietnam.

Appendix D

E. Coli Assessment

Some comments[1] by Edmund Crouch, PhD, Cambridge Environmental Inc.
to the
Second Meeting of the
Committee on the Review of the Draft USDA *E. coli* O157:H7
Farm-to-Table Process Risk Assessment
Monday, December 17, 2001

Author's note to the reader:
These remarks were originally prepared after the IOM committee requested that I comment on the implementation of the E. coli *risk assessment model and they have not been peer-reviewed. Some minor editorial changes have been made from the version of the paper submitted to the committee. The remarks address the draft model contained in the spreadsheet "ECRA 010801-a.xls," dated August 8, 2001. They were specifically written for an audience who had ready access to the draft USDA risk assessment and spreadsheet, and it will be difficult for anyone who does not have these documents to understand them.*

GENERAL

I was requested to examine in particular the implementation of the model described in this Risk Assessment, so the following concentrates on the spreadsheet, although unavoidably I have to comment on other matters as well.

There is some evidence that the spreadsheet provided to the committee is not the spreadsheet that was actually used to provide results in the document, but one in the stages of being modified to something different (perhaps to incorporate other functions, and/or other studies). The evidence lies in:

---

[1] These comments were requested by the committee, which paid my expenses to present them. Some of my time writing these comments was paid for by Cambridge Environmental Inc., but the majority was unfunded.

1. Compilation errors. The VBA code would not compile as supplied (see below, under "VBA code"). Some of the compilation errors looked as though they were occurring because what was provided was a work in progress (e.g., possible modifications in progress).

2. Cross-referencing errors in the spreadsheet. See the sections on the "BreedingHerds" and "Feedlots" sheets under "Herd prevalence": studies used do not match those documented. These cross-referencing errors could have been introduced during an update that was adding/modifying studies.

SOME IMPLEMENTATION ISSUES

Notation

In what follows, an unqualified page number refers to the *E. coli* risk assessment, PDF version. I occasionally refer to a page number in Appendix C, but I am then explicit (and the page number might be slightly different from other copies, because Appendix C is in Word, so page numbers depend slightly on printer type).

References within spreadsheets are generally given in A1 notation. The sheet name is also given (e.g., SlaughterData!F39) if the sheet reference is not the sheet that is currently under discussion (i.e., is not the current section heading).

Documentation in Appendix C

"It was decided to use specific cell references rather than named ranges throughout the workbook. Although this makes changes to the model more difficult to accomplish, it should make it easier to follow and audit the flow in the procedures."

This is contrary to my experience, in particular with this program, but also in general, and contrary to discussions of programming methods of which I am aware. This implementation is poorly documented and difficult to follow. The statement quoted is especially unusual since the default method of cell labeling (A1 style, letter column followed by numbered row) that is used in the documentation does not correspond to the method used within Visual Basic for Applications (VBA). In VBA, the preferred method of cell reference (and that used in much of, perhaps all, the programming here) is an entry like "cell(14,3)", which means the cell at row 14 and column 3. This corresponds to the alternative labeling method in Excel, called R1C1 style, where a cell is referenced by row number and column number (i.e., the reverse order to the default, and using numbers for both row and column). Thus one has to get used to and translate be-

APPENDIX D

tween a labeling style that is not the default, and is in reverse order to standard Cartesian axis labeling.

As an example of the problems, the following are said to be uncertainty distributions. Without some translation, I find this list uninformative. Trying to compare with the VBA code SimUncertainty (where the cell references are given in the cell(row,col) form) presents considerable difficulty. Here are some translations.

Feedlots!C31	Oct.–May herd prevalence
Feedlots!C32	June-Sept. herd prevalence
Feedlots!F33	Herd prevalence (not season-specific)
BreedingHerds!C31	Oct.–May herd prevalence
BreedingHerds!C32	June-Sept. herd prevalence
BreedingHerds!F33	Herd prevalence (not season-specific)
SlaughterData!E8	Carcass prevalence/fecal prevalence (summer)
SlaughterData!G8	Carcass prevalence/fecal prevalence (winter)
SlaughterData!C78	
SlaughterData!C81	
SlaughterData!C83	
SlaughterData!C88	
SlaughterData!C92	
SlaughterData!E12	Trim/Vacuum/Wash, most likely decontamination
SlaughterData!F12	Trim/Vacuum/Wash, maximum decontamination
SlaughterData!D15	Evisceration, probability of rupture
SlaughterData!E20	Steam pasteurization, most likely decontamination
SlaughterData!F20	Steam pasteurization, maximum decontamination
SlaughterData!D22	
SlaughterData!L29	
SlaughterData!L30	
SlaughterData!L31	
SlaughterData!F38	
SlaughterData!F39	
SlaughterData!F40	
SlaughterData!G25	
SlaughterData!G26	
GrowthData!C6:E6	

GrowthData!F13:H22
GrowthData!M8:M21
GrowthData!J22
GrowthData!P22
GrowthData!B26

Cooking!O7:O15
Cooking!J20
Cooking!K20
Cooking!G59

DR!M2

VBA Code

Compilation

Attempting to compile the VBA code resulted in the following errors.

Module RunSegments; Subroutine GrowthOnly
sGrinder not defined
sCoreModelBook not defined
sResultsBook not defined

Module Functions; Function SortString
When @Risk is not loaded, the built-in VBA function Mid is not recognized unless all references to @Risk are removed (for example, on the Tools:References list in the VBA editor). Similarly, other string functions (e.g., Left) are not recognized in similar circumstances. This behavior is odd, and may indicate that @Risk is doing something odd. However, it may simply be a bug in the behavior of the VBA compiler when it has unresolved external references (it is a bug because it is falsely signaling an error).

Module Functions; Function TrapezoidInv
dMidArea not defined
mean not defined
pMid2 incomplete statement
TriangInv incorrectly referenced (multiple times)
pMid not defined
plus many more.

It was necessary to "comment out" this entire routine to get compilation.

Module FullRun, Subroutine RunGrowthOnly
  sUncertFilt not defined
  sUncertainty not defined

Module X NotUsed, Subroutine SimulateAll
  Call to subroutine MultiSimSlaughter not defined

Questions On The Code

Module Uncertainty. Subroutine SimUncertainty.
Why does this recalculate the Uncertainty sheet every 20 iterations of the i loop? This appears superfluous, and simply slows the calculation.

BREEDING HERDS SHEET

1. Herd prevalence: studies used do not match those documented.

At page 38 (just above Equation 3.4) it is stated that "True breeding herd prevalence (Figure 3-2) was estimated by combining the results from Equation 3.2 across all seven studies using Equation 3.4." The seven studies referred to are in Table 3-1 on page 36. The spreadsheet model lists 10 studies (columns C:L), of which the first 7 are used in the estimate (columns P:V reference columns C:I). These are not the 7 studies in Table 3-1. The effect is to omit the studies labeled as Hancock et al., 1998; Lagreid et al., 1999; and Hancock et al., 1997a in Table 3-1 (taking account of the different names assigned in the spreadsheet). The extra studies included have no effect—they are included with zero entries that lead to likelihoods of unity.

Some columns in the spreadsheet match these experiments (with minor changes in attributed dates), but the entries that are used for computation do not, as illustrated in the following tables:

Table 3-1	Spreadsheet	Column
Hancock et al., 1997a	Hancock, 1997a	I
Hancock et al., 1997b	Hancock, 1997b	L
Hancock et al., 1998a	Hancock, 1998	J
Garber et al., 1999	Garber, 1998	C
Lagreid et al., 1999	Lagreid, 1998	K
Sargeant et al., 2000	Sargeant, 2000	G
Hancock, 2001	Hancock/FDA, 2001	H

As used in spreadsheet

Column Name	Column	Column Referenced	Study Referenced
Garber, 1998	P	C	Garber, 1999
Hancock, 1997a	Q	D	Besser, 1997 (null)
Hancock, 1998	R	E	Rice, 1997 (null)
Lagreid, 1998	S	F	Hancock, 1994 (null)
Hancock, 1997b	T	G	Sargeant, 2000
Sargeant, 2000	U	H	Hancock, 2001
Hancock/FDA, 2001 (7)	V	I	Hancock, 1997a

Entries listed as (null) have no entries in the relevant columns, and contribute no variation to the likelihood. Thus the spreadsheet headings do not match internally, nor with Table 3-1 (page 36).

This confusion presumably originally arose because of the additional information included in the spreadsheet at I3, that some studies did not include the sampling of adult cattle.

2. The method of application of Bayes theorem is crude. There are much better options available.

The aim was to find a distribution of probabilities (between 0 and 1). The method adopted was to compute the likelihood for increments of 0.01 in probability (between 0.01 and 1 inclusive; 0 necessarily has zero likelihood), then return a random variate with discrete values (integer multiples of 0.01) with probability proportional to the likelihood. This replaces a continuous variate with a discrete one, and may possibly produce odd effects in some simulations—e.g., we have no idea about the random number generator used; it is possible that one could get an interaction with the structure of the random number generator.

A better approach is to design a generator that produces random variates with a distribution function proportional to the likelihood—in the notation of Equation 3.2, page 37, all that is required is a generator with distribution function proportional to

$$\prod_{i=1}^{4} (Hsens_i \times \Phi)^{S_i} (1 - Hsens_i \times \Phi)^{N_i - S_i}$$

where i labels the different sets of observations. This is relatively straightforward. For example, this distribution should be amenable to processing using a "universal" method of random number generation (see e.g., UNURAN at http://statistik.wu-wien.ac.at/unuran/).

APPENDIX D   153

3. The method of calculation of the combined likelihood is unnecessarily complicated, and unnecessarily slows the computations.

The implementation proceeds in stages, appending each experiment one after the other. At each stage, a binomial term (see Equation 3.2, page 37) is computed (by a call to a built-in Excel function BINOMDIST, columns P:V) for each of the 100 values of probability (0.01 step 0.01 to 1.00, column O) . Then the likelihood is updated by multiplying by the binomial term, and the result is re-normalized. All the renormalization steps are unnecessary. All the binomial calculations unnecessarily include the computation of a "combination" term ($^{N}C_{S}$) that is relatively expensive (time-consuming) to compute (this is internal to the BINOMDIST function). All that is required is the product given by the equation above. The final normalization is not necessary, because the RiskDiscrete function subsequently used (at F33) performs such a normalization internally (this feature is apparently undocumented, but is essential for such a function).

4. The values of *Hsens* used in the computations do not match the values given in the documentation.

The values for *Hsens* for Breeding Herds are listed on page 38. The values used in the spreadsheets differ. The values are (rounded to 2 significant figures):

Experiment	Documentation	Spreadsheet (P2:V2)
Garber et al., 1999	0.75	0.75
Lagreid et al., 1999	0.86	not used
Sargeant et al., 2000	0.86	0.99
Hancock et al., 1998a	0.89	not used
Hancock, 2001	0.89	0.87
Hancock et al., 1997b	0.96	not used
Hancock et al., 1997a	0.99	0.89

This is undoubtedly because of the mix-up already described above.

5. The uncertainty of Herd Sensitivity (page 37, symbol *Hsens*) is ignored.

The uncertainty in the estimate of *Hsens* is considerable. None of that uncertainty is propagated into the calculations. *Hsens* is fixed (it is listed in P2:V2)—and the VBA code setting up uncertainty estimates does not alter this fixed value.

6. The calculation of *Hsens* appears to be incorrect.

The calculation method for *Hsens* is simply described as "using Monte Carlo methods" (page 38, first paragraph), so we cannot be sure what was done. However, the spreadsheet contains a calculation of a quantity called "Herd sensitivity" (at C12:L12). Equation 3.3 on page 37 defines *Hsens* as

$$Hsens = 1 - \int (1 - p)^n f(p) dp$$

where p is the "apparent within-herd prevalence," f(p) is the "frequency" of p, and n is the number of animals tested in a herd. No limits were specified for the integral. Apparent within-herd prevalence is then said to be exponentially distributed between herds (pages 39–41), and proportional to the true prevalence (page 43, Equation 3.5). Let η be the test sensitivity and q the true within-herd prevalence, with distribution across herds g(q). Then

$$Hsens = 1 - \int_0^1 (1 - \eta q)^n g(q) dq$$
$$= 1 - \int_0^\eta (1 - p)^n f(p) dp$$

If f is exponential with parameter β (page 39, last paragraph), it must necessarily be a truncated exponential (so that its mean and standard deviation are not quite β, contrary to page 39). Examination of the spreadsheet entries at C12:L12 (in the row labeled "Herd sensitivity") shows a formula equivalent to

$$Hsens(?) = 1 - (1 - p)^n$$

where the "?" has been added because it is not clear what is being calculated here, even though it is labeled "Herd sensitivity." This formula is clearly different from the "Herd sensitivity" listed in the documentation. However, this value does not appear to be used anywhere in the spreadsheets, although presumably it may have been used to evaluate the values used for Hsens in a subsidiary calculation. Otherwise, these entries are unnecessary, misleading, and simply serve to slow down the spreadsheet calculation.

7. The method of application of the Test Sensitivity is incorrect.

Test sensitivity is discussed at page 43, and used as in Equation 3.5. Obviously, Equation 3.5 can be correct only so long as "apparent prevalence" is lower than the test sensitivity. However, in the spreadsheet, the

APPENDIX D   155

impossible situation of "apparent prevalence" higher than "test sensitivity" is handled incorrectly (see, for example, F24).

It appears that the methodology attempted in the spreadsheet is based on likelihood methods (this is explicit for "true herd prevalence" Φ, and implicit for other parameters where uncertainty distributions for binomial observations are taken to be beta distributions). In fact, it appears that an attempt is being made to draw samples from conditional likelihoods—hence the conditioning of the distribution for Φ on the herd sensitivity, for example.

At F24, the equation used is MIN(RiskBeta(2+1,84−2+1)/$F$15,1). The RiskBeta function samples from a beta distribution corresponding to a binomial observation, and the result is divided by a test sensitivity that is itself a sample drawn from a beta distribution, again based on a binomial distribution. The impossible situation of the "apparent prevalence" higher than the "test sensitivity" is handled by substituting unity for the ratio, but the correct approach to obtain a sample distribution proportional to the conditional likelihood is to censor this sample combination, not to arbitrarily replace it. The effect of the replacement performed is to drastically distort the uncertainty distribution. The information on test sensitivity provided by the field study is being rejected, and instead replaced with some other (undefined) assumption.

Similar problems arise for all the estimates of seasonal prevalence. Note that the MIN function has only been applied in the spreadsheet to the Hancock (1994) study. Presumably that is the only one where the field study provides any real extra information about the test sensitivity. (The apparent prevalence is too rarely higher than the test sensitivity in the other cases to ever have arisen in any of the samples, or such cases were not noticed.)

<u>8. Table 3-4 and associated text and calculations are undocumented and possibly incorrect.</u>

The origin of the frequency distribution in Table 3-4 is not documented. The symbol x used in the text is clearly supposed to be the concentration (not the $\log_{10}$ of the concentration) of CFU/gram, so that the usual meaning of f(x) would be the distribution function for the concentration of CFU/gram, not the distribution function for $\log_{10}$(CFU/gram). In that case the calculations performed in Table 3-4 are incorrect, because they ignore the non-linear (indeed, logarithmic) scale of CFU/gram on the left (as does the normalization of f(x)). More likely, f(x) is supposed to represent the distribution function for $\log_{10}$(CFU/gram). Even then, the sum calculated probably does not adequately represent the required calculation, because of the high non-linearity in the exponential term being averaged.

9. At least one test sensitivity used does not agree with the documented value.

The study of Hancock (1994) is documented (page 45) as using 0.1-gram samples and TSBv-SMAC. This is estimated on page 45 to have a test sensitivity of 2%. The value used in the spreadsheet has an expected value of 7.7%, almost 4 times higher. The calculation (cell C38) leading to this higher estimate is not documented.

10. There is no evidence for "seasonal variability" presented in the documentation.

"Examining the monthly prevalence evidence, there appears to be a high prevalence season (June to September) and a low prevalence season (October to May)." (Page 45). The only evidence presented is: "For example, Garber et al. (1999) sampled cattle from February through July. These data show that 7 of 193 cattle sampled in infected herds were fecal positive during the period from February to May. In contrast, 44 of 1,075 cattle sampled in infected herds during June and July were fecal positive." This is not a contrast, however—the rates presented could hardly be more similar ($p = 0.47$, one-sided Fisher exact test). The only other study with results known separately for sampling in these two periods is Hancock/FDA (2001), showing 15/2,831 in December through March, versus 23/2,878 in June through September (documented only in a spreadsheet comment. This shows a larger contrast in rates, but again there is no significant difference ($p = 0.11$, one-sided Fisher exact test).

The only evidence for seasonal difference in prevalence appears to come from comparisons between different studies, although this evidence was not discussed. The difference is most apparent between Hancock (1994) (performed only in summer) and the other studies. However, the prevalence estimate in Hancock (1994), is highly inflated by the estimated test sensitivity (and maybe should be inflated more—see above). Moreover, this study contains very few animals compared with the others. An adequate test for difference in seasonal variability needs to be carried out.

11. The method for averaging within-herd prevalence over "seasons" necessarily mixes any true seasonal difference with between-study differences.

The method adopted for obtaining seasonal averages of within-herd prevalence appears to be ad hoc. Were complete-year data available for every study, the imputations implied in the method adopted necessarily would reduce any seasonal differences that exist. Each study is imputed to have tested equal numbers of animals in every month of the study, and, where explicit time-resolved data are not available, the within-herd prevalence for every month for which aggregate data are available is assumed to be equal. For example, for Besser (1997), the aggregate results over 12 months were known to be 53 positives in 2,074. This rate was assumed to apply for each month (e.g., see D19:D30). The first imputation (equal numbers of animals) is perhaps plausible; but the second (equal rates in all seasons) is contrary to the assumption of the analysis. If there is any contrast between seasons, the second imputation forces the analysis to underestimate it.

On the other hand, since some studies provide information only within particular months, and there are possibly substantial differences between studies in the same months, the method adopted necessarily confounds seasonal differences with study differences.

It would be straightforward to perform a likelihood analysis that makes an assumption of different rates in different months. However, in view of the lack of any evidence of contrast between seasons, this appears unnecessary. Almost the entire "seasonal" difference indicated in the documentation is due to the inclusion of the high values from Hancock (1994), even though that has low weight. But the values obtained in Hancock et al. (1994) are highly skewed by a highly uncertain test sensitivity value (see previous comments).

FEEDLOTS

Most or all of the problems discussed above for the BreedingHerds sheet also occur in the Feedlots sheet. I only mention a few of them here, for example, to give the spreadsheet references (they usually differ from the BreedingHerds references).

<u>12. Herd prevalence: studies used do not match those documented.</u>

As for BreedingHerds, there is a mismatch between documentation and spreadsheet. The documentation says that Dargatz et al., 1997; Hancock et al., 1998b; Smith, 1999; and Elder et al., 2000, were used (page 48, and Table 3-6). These correspond to columns C, E, F, and G. There is an additional "Hancock 1999" in column D. However, the columns concatenated are C, D, E, and F. The effect is to omit Elder et al., 2000 (the erroneously included "Hancock 1999" has zero entries that contribute a constant to the likelihood).

13. The values of *Hsens* used in the computations do not match the values given in the documentation.

The values for *Hsens* for feedlots are listed on page 48. The values used in the spreadsheets differ. The values are (rounded to 2 significant figures):

	Page 48	Spreadsheet
Dargatz et al., 1997	0.77	0.75
Hancock et al., 1998b	0.86	0.99 (labeled as Smith, 1999, in column N)
Smith, 1999	0.99	0.81 (labeled as Elder, 2000, in column O)
Elder et al., 2000	0.81	This reference not used in the spreadsheet.

This is undoubtedly because of the mix-up already described above.

14. The uncertainty of *Hsens* is ignored.

Hsens is fixed (it is listed in L2:O2).

SLAUGHTERDATA SHEET

15. The distributions for several quantities are not justified.

At pages 65–66, we have "the reduction from decontamination (D1) was modeled using a triangular distribution with a minimum value of 0 logs, an uncertain most likely value ranging from 0.3 to 0.7 logs, and an uncertain maximum value ranging from 0.8 logs to 1.2 logs." In fact, although not specified here, the two uncertainty ranges given were used to define uncorrelated uniform distributions. See E12, F12, SlaughterXXModel!I16 and SlaughterXXModel!K16 where XX is CB or SH. No basis whatever is given for selecting uniform distributions for the uncertainty, nor for selecting a triangular distribution for the variability distribution.

Other similar distributions occur at various places, all without justification. For example, see page 67, steam pasteurization in the second decontamination (step 5). In the spreadsheet, this is at E20, F20, and SlaughterXXModel!K16 where XX is CB or SH. Similarly for the chiller (step 6), at page 67, where we have a "normal distribution with an uncertain mean ranging from –0.5 to 0.5 logs and a standard deviation of 1 log."

The spreadsheet uses a uniform for the mean (see D22 and SlaughterXXModel!F10 where XX is CB or SH).

16. Small plant, second decontamination (wash). Ambiguous documentation, and implementation that differs from any recognized interpretation.

Page 67: "It was assumed that small plants typically use a hot water rinse, sometimes supplemented with organic acids. The effectiveness of hot water rinsing is assumed equivalent to that described for decontamination Step 1 (D1)."

The meaning of this statement is ambiguous. What does "equivalent" mean—is the effectiveness of hot water rinsing within a given plant assumed to be identical to D1 for that plant, or to be equal in probability to D1 for that plant, or something else? What was implemented was equality in probability. The spreadsheet takes the same values for the "most likely" and "maximum" log reductions from their uncertainty distributions, but implements the variability distributions through separate instances of triangular distributions.

A FEW OTHER SPECIFIC COMMENTS

Page 18, para –2
In Washington state... The numbers have switched somewhere. 13/445 is 2.9%, and 5/445 is 1.1%, but these are cited as the other way round.

Page 43, last para
10^7 in what units?

Page 43, last para
"A minimum shedding concentration of 10^{-1} colony-forming units (CFU) per gram of feces can be assumed, based on a 10-gram sample." What is the evidence for this statement? That may be the detection limit, but it does not necessarily correspond to the lowest possible concentration.

Page 44
"Therefore, the observed difference in sensitivity between these methods approximates the effect of different sample quantities." Is this proposed as a justification for f(x) in Table 3-4? It isn't.

Page 44 and page 45
"Yet a 1.0-gram sample from infected cattle is only 85% likely to contain *E. coli* O157:H7." "A 0.1-gram sample from infected cattle is only 73%

likely to contain *E. coli* O157:H7." These statements apparently rely on Table 3-4, for which no evidence is presented.

Page 45

Hancock et al. (1994) sampling was estimated to have only 2% sensitivity, yet they detected 4.4% positive. And the difference is statistically significant even if the herd is 100% infected (p = 0.001). There is something wrong with this estimate. Also, equation 3.5 then predicts more than 100% prevalence, an impossibility. See the discussion of the BreedingHerds sheet.

Page 55, Equation 3.6

This represents a documentation failure, and a failure (at least in the documentation) to realize obvious speedups. The random variate B generated by this complicated sum is simply Binomial(40,H^*w) as it is written. What the writers intended to say was that w is selected from an exponential variability distribution on each variability iteration, or something of that nature. The spreadsheet removes the unnecessary summation.

Page 56, Equation 3.7

Same problem. Again, the spreadsheet removes the unnecessary summation.

Page 61

"individual carcass contributes (n) ranged from 2 to 6. In cow/bull plants, this range was 2 to 4. Uncertainty about the most likely number of combo bins per carcass was modeled as a uniform(2,5) and uniform(2,3) for steer/heifer and cow/bull plants, respectively. The ranges and most likely values were modeled using triangular (min, most likely, max) distributions." These three sentences all contradict one another, the first two as to numbers, the second two as to distributions assumed. And none gives any evidentiary basis for the selections.

Page 62, Equation 3.9

It is not clear whether the number of truckloads should be an integer, or this is estimating the average number of truckloads.

Page 63, high and low prevalence seasons for TR

(a) Why is the approach taken for estimating TR different for the high and low seasons?

(b) Such measurements as are discussed suggest that there is a nonlinear effect here—at low prevalence TR is less than unity; at high prevalence, it is higher than unity. However, the modeling completely ignores

APPENDIX D   161

this nonlinearity. But it might be very important to include it. It is stated that "more uncertainty is modeled about TR during this season"—but that is not what the discussed measurements indicate. The Bacon et al. (2000) measurements showing lower TR appear to have been entirely ignored—there is no discussion of their uncertainty.

(c) It is not stated here what is meant by a "a mixture of the beta distributions based on the Elder et al. (2000) data and a uniform distribution with a minimum approaching 0 and a maximum of the summer TR." What is done in the spreadsheet is to use a 50% probability mixture between the ratio of betas and a uniform ranging from zero to that ratio. No evidence is presented that such a mixture provides a good representation of the uncertainty involved.